HOW TO PREPARE FOR

Medical School

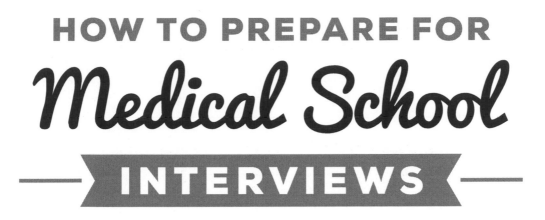

INTERVIEWS

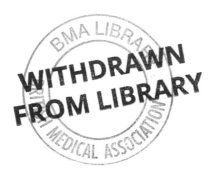

Philip McElnay

NIHR Academic Clinical Fellow and
Cardiothoracic Surgery Specialist Trainee

Scion

© **Scion Publishing Limited, 2016**

First published 2016

A CIP catalogue record for this book is available from the British Library.

ISBN 978 1 907904 83 7

Scion Publishing Limited

The Old Hayloft, Vantage Business Park, Bloxham Road, Banbury OX16 9UX, UK
www.scionpublishing.com

Important Note from the Publisher

The information contained within this book was obtained by Scion Publishing Ltd from sources believed by us to be reliable. However, while every effort has been made to ensure its accuracy, no responsibility for loss or injury whatsoever occasioned to any person acting or refraining from action as a result of information contained herein can be accepted by the authors or publishers.

Readers are reminded that medicine is a constantly evolving science and while the authors and publishers have ensured that all dosages, applications and practices are based on current indications, there may be specific practices which differ between communities. You should always follow the guidelines laid down by the manufacturers of specific products and the relevant authorities in the country in which you are practising.

Although every effort has been made to ensure that all owners of copyright material have been acknowledged in this publication, we would be pleased to acknowledge in subsequent reprints or editions any omissions brought to our attention.

Registered names, trademarks, etc. used in this book, even when not marked as such, are not to be considered unprotected by law.

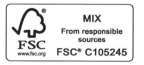

Typeset by Medlar Publishing Solutions Pvt Ltd, India
Printed in the UK

Contents

List of contributors

Saima Azam	University College London
Shreya Badhrinarayanan	Brighton and Sussex Medical School
Ali Bakhsh	Peninsula College of Medicine and Dentistry
Michael F. Bath	University of Leicester
Gayathri Bhaskaran	Barts and the London
Oliver Brewster	University of Cambridge
Scott Colvin	University of Glasgow
Natalia Cotton	University of Oxford
Praveena Deekonda	University of Exeter
Reema Gardner	University of Warwick
Cathal Hannan	Queen's University Belfast
Cara Jenvey	University of Keele
Khalid Khan	University of Nottingham
Chetan Khatri	Imperial College London
Mehreen Mahfooz	University of Leeds
Ashish Mandavia	University of Bristol
Annika Mills	Swansea University
Midhun Mohan	University of Liverpool
Kiran Nadeem	University of Manchester
Thomas Parsons	University College London
Anna Porter	Newcastle University
Emma Rengasamy	Cardiff University
Amy Szuman	Hull York Medical School
Ben Williamson	King's College London

Foreword

Being a doctor is rewarding. You care for people when they are at their most vulnerable, and on occasion they may even be entrusting their very lives to you. Being a doctor is exciting. There are few careers which see you frequently intervene to improve someone's quality or quantity of life.

Being a doctor can be challenging. It is a busy career with lots to learn and lots of demands made on your energy, time and emotions. However, you will rarely find a doctor who does not relish turning up on the ward, at the operating theatre or the surgery every morning – it's a privilege.

But it shouldn't be a career just for the privileged. A healthy health service has a spectrum of healthcare professionals from all backgrounds. Medicine thrives on innovation and the ability of its practitioners to empathise with people from every walk of life.

One of the biggest hurdles in pursuing a career in medicine is getting that coveted place at medical school. Just because the position is coveted, however, should not mean it is reserved for those who have inside knowledge of the process or are well connected enough to be coached through the predictable medical school interview questions.

Books such as this can help overcome that barrier, and clearly explain the process of applying to medical school and preparing for your interview. Be proud if you have got that far – and see your interview as your opportunity to showcase your ability, your personality and your enthusiasm for a career in medicine. If you haven't started applying yet don't let the competition put you off – the challenge is worth it for a lifelong career that is rewarding, exciting and challenging.

Good luck – you can do it!

Professor Sir Norman Williams

Director of the National Centre for Bowel Research and Surgical Innovation
Barts & the London School of Medicine & Dentistry
Queen Mary, University of London

March 2016

Preface

"Do you come from a medical family?" is a question that any medical student or junior doctor will empathise with.

I'm unsure why, but medics have traditionally seemed to breed medics, and they make fantastic doctors.

However, I am a passionate believer that those who don't come from medical families make equally fantastic doctors. Not better. Not worse. Equally fantastic.

And it was with that equality in mind that I and twenty equally fantastic medics set about creating this book. I've worked with some absolutely wonderful medical students and doctors from almost every medical school in the UK. Our aim was to consolidate the conversations, tips and preparation advice that anyone could have if they chatted to a consultant physician or surgeon about applying to medical school. Some applicants know those people. Some don't. But whether you are the son or daughter of a brain surgeon, engineer, plumber, psychiatrist, GP or shop assistant I hope this book helps provide that information.

Whether your mum or dad are phenomenally well connected, or you no longer know them, if you want to apply to medical school you should do it. It doesn't matter what background you're from. If you have the skill, ability and caring nature to be a doctor, you should be a doctor. I sincerely hope that this book can help demystify the process of getting there, and put you on an equal footing to be an equally fantastic doctor.

Good luck and believe in yourself.

#WideningParticipation
#WideningAccess

Philip McElnay
@phil_mce

March 2016

Chapter 1 |
Applications and interview preparation

Applying to medical school is a slightly different process to applying to study most other subjects. Applications are made through UCAS but almost all medical courses have an earlier deadline for submission: start planning well in advance! Depending on which courses you apply to, you may have to take the UK Clinical Aptitude Test (**UKCAT** – www.ukcat. ac.uk), BioMedical Admissions Test (**BMAT** – www.admissionstestingservice.org/for-test-takers/bmat/) or both. These tests are designed to distinguish between the best applicants in the country and have an unusual format, so preparation is essential.

The majority of medical schools will then consider your application and create a shortlist to invite for interview. Offers will be based on all the information that they have received: exam grades, UKCAT/BMAT results, personal statement and interview scores. There are some important exceptions, which do not routinely interview UK school leavers. This is always subject to change and we recommend you read the online prospectus of your chosen universities well in advance.

Each medical school puts different weighting on certain aspects of the application. Some choose candidates entirely on the basis of the UKCAT, some use a GCSE grade cut-off and some interview almost everyone. They are transparent about their interview selection procedure and it is worth working out the aspects of your application that are strongest and choosing universities that rate them highly.

Personal statements are important for two reasons. Firstly, they form the only really individual part of your electronic application (most medical school applicants have broadly similar grades and test results). Secondly, during your interview you can expect to be asked about specific details and must be prepared to defend, elaborate upon or discuss them.

Interviews vary widely between medical schools, ranging from a scientific cross-examination to a 15-minute chat about empathy and motivation. Many universities are employing a new format of interview with multiple stations including short traditional interviews as well as tasks and challenges. These are termed Multiple Mini Interviews (MMIs). Once again, whether your chosen university uses this format can usually be gleaned from the internet.

Offers are usually sent in letter or email form. They can arrive late in the day: don't let this stress you out! Some medical schools will invite offer holders to a second open day, which can help you to decide where to rank each offer.

Graduate applicants

Graduate applicants to medicine come from a variety of backgrounds.

One of the biggest barriers to graduates attending medical school may be financial, but support is out there. National student finance agencies have a range of funding options and there are charities, loans, scholarships and bursaries that can assist graduates.

A number of institutions offer accelerated four-year programmes for graduates. This allows for the completion of the course in a shorter, but more intense, timeframe. Traditional five- or six-year courses also still accept graduates.

Applications are also processed through UCAS and institutions still employ a variety of entrance exams including the UKCAT and BMAT.

Anecdotally, graduates may perform better at interview but expectations are high. A variety of interview techniques are also utilised, from traditional panel interview to a multiple mini interview format.

About the Multiple Mini Interview (MMI)

Questions in MMI format are indicated by '(MMI)' beside the question number in this book.

What are MMIs?

MMI stations are designed to test a range of skills. They involve a number of different, short interviews or role-play scenarios. For example, you may be given one minute to read a set of instructions outside a room. A whistle may then be blown and you will enter the room to perform the task. You will be given a set amount of time to perform the task, e.g. 7 minutes. At the end of the 7 minutes (often with a warning whistle at 6 minutes) a whistle may be blown again and you will rotate to the next station, having one minute to read the brief outside the station again. This will continue for multiple stations, e.g. ten stations. There will be interviewers who will mark your performance in each station and a decision will be taken on your overall performance. Often there will be a number of staff outside the interview rooms to guide you around the circuit.

The stations will often involve challenging and unfamiliar scenarios. Interviewers are eager to assess whether you will be able to communicate effectively in a range of situations, as well as being able to follow instructions, rationally consider complex problems and display a range of technical skills.

The questions may require a small amount of medical knowledge (i.e. enough to demonstrate that you have an interest in medicine) but on the whole they are designed to allow you to demonstrate the range of skills described above without being a medical expert. After being given a written or verbal brief before the station you will often be asked to communicate with an actor or the interviewer in the station.

How do I practise?

The key to success in these scenarios (and in traditional interviews!) is to practise frequently before the interview – you can use this book as a starting point. Pair up with a friend or family member. Ask them to be the actor/interviewer in the scenario and to read the answer in order to develop the situation appropriately. You, as the candidate, should read the brief provided in the question (and no more!) and then speak to your friend as if you are in the real interview. Allow them to develop the scenario as described in the answer. Ask them to provide feedback to you.

Some key tips

If you are asked to communicate with someone in station there are some key concepts that will be common to each scenario. Whilst we don't have room to mention them each time in the answer you should consider doing each of the following things if the station asks you to talk to someone:

Introduce yourself – the brief will often tell you who you are playing: *"Hello, my name is John and I am a medical student"*.

Start with open questions – *"Can you tell me a little bit about why you are here today?"* as opposed to closed questions such as *"Where is your pain?"*

Summarise your conversation at the end of the station – *"Just to check I have got everything clear in my mind – your computer broke last week, you brought it to us for repair and you are unhappy with the service we have provided"*.

Conclude the conversation – *"Thank you for coming to see me today; I will raise what we have discussed with my supervisor and come back to you today with a solution. See you soon"*. Perhaps offer a handshake, if it feels comfortable!

About the traditional interview

> **Questions in traditional format are denoted by '(T)' beside the question number in this book.**

Many medical schools across the UK have embraced the MMI format to conduct their interviews. There are a number, however, that still conduct a single, formal 'across the table'-style interview, with applicants being asked questions by a number of interviewers. Sometimes this format of questioning is used in an MMI station too (and some of the content from the MMI questions contained in this book can also find their way into traditional-style interviews) – don't forget to prepare both styles of questions.

The questions asked might range from queries about extra-curricular activities to something you mentioned in your UCAS personal statement. The interviewers may debate medical politics with you, delve into your reasons for applying or seek to test your scientific knowledge. Regardless of the strength of your application, preparation for this style of interview is important. In fact, both MMI and traditional interview preparation is likened in quantity and intensity to that for an exam!

TOP TIPS

- Start preparing early – get a friend or family member to ask you questions from this book and answer them as if you were in an interview.
- Speak to junior doctors, consultants, GPs, current medical students (especially those at the medical school to which you are applying) – ask them about the things they love about their job (or the course), but also quiz them about the challenges. Don't forget to mention to the interviewer that you have done this.
- At least a week before, prepare what you are going to wear. Unless your invitation to interview tells you otherwise, you must look impeccable. Despite male doctors infrequently wearing ties now, males should still wear a shirt, suit and tie. Don't forget to polish your shoes.
- Arrange/book your travel well in advance and allow some contingency time in case of road works, train delays, poor weather, etc.
- Smile! And practise smiling! By demonstrating that you are approachable and friendly you will make a much better impression than if you appear glum and nervous. It might be difficult to smile, and you will be nervous, but smiling can actually give you confidence and may even make the interviewer smile back, which will give you even more confidence!
- Arrange work experience – find out if medicine is for you. Speak to hospitals, GP practices, private hospitals, nursing homes; people will want to help you. If at first you find it difficult to arrange work experience, keep trying – you may need to be persistent but always be very polite!
- If you have been invited to interview: congratulations! This is a huge achievement in itself and you have clearly impressed the medical school already. Medicine needs a huge variety of people and you should believe in your own abilities without being arrogant. Good luck!

Chapter 2 | Applying to Oxford or Cambridge

Applying to Oxford or Cambridge may be daunting but if you'd like to go you should definitely apply! Have the courage to believe that you could get in no matter how remote a possibility it might feel.

Start thinking early about how to structure your personal statement, as this often guides the interviewers' questions. Before your interview, research areas of interest that you can talk about fluently and articulately – for example, the Ebola outbreak or new break-throughs in Alzheimer's disease research – as you may be asked if there's a topic you'd like to discuss during the interview.

Cambridge and Oxford both use a college-based university system and it is worth reading about this online before your interview. Often colleges set up one academic and one non-academic interview, so don't forget to brush up on your answers to the common non-academic questions listed in this book. Some colleges are in higher demand than others and the competition ratios can vary. Oxford and Cambridge have different systems to combat this effect and ensure that the best students get a place at the university no matter which college they apply to. In Oxford you will be allocated an interview at a second college. If you get offers from both colleges, then the college you originally applied to gets priority. In Cambridge you only interview for the college you apply to, but the highest-ranking unsuccessful candidates are placed in a 'pool' and can be selected by other colleges that year. The colleges that select out of the pool can either give an offer straight away or interview the candidate again.

Be prepared to be unprepared. Up until now, it is likely that you will have entered exams and similar scenarios with a pretty good idea of what is likely to come up. However, the whole basis and aim of the Oxbridge interview is to take you outside your comfort zone and encourage you to really think. I can almost guarantee that there will be questions to which you don't know the answer and have never even considered before. The vital thing here is to accept this before you go to interview, and not to let it intimidate you. It will be the same for every other interviewee. The interview is not a simple knowledge test, but rather an opportunity for you to demonstrate how you are able to apply basic principles in unfamiliar scenarios and handle pressure: both are vital skills for any future doctor. Have a look at *Chapter 10* to gain more experience of how to answer very unfamiliar questions.

Finally, be enthusiastic! Oxbridge academics meet their students regularly for small tutorials, so they use the interviews to decide whether they feel you would benefit from this sort of interaction and if you would fit in. Your interviewers may ask questions on the subjects that most interest them and if you clearly enjoy discussing and learning about science it will go a long way. Practise spontaneous and stretching conversations about science with your science teachers or friends.

Believe in yourself, and good luck.

Chapter 3 | Questions about you

3.1 (T) What skills or characteristics do you possess that would make you fit in in a problem-based learning group?

This is a question asking you to outline the skills that you possess. It is a good idea to start an answer to skills-based questions with a broad sentence such as:

"I believe I would be an active and effective member of a PBL group for a number of reasons:"

and then, giving three or four skills in a structured manner makes you sound considered and logical, i.e. *"Firstly,... Secondly,... and finally,...".*

When describing a skill you possess, back it up with an example and explain how it would make you an ideal medical student. For example:

"Firstly, I have very good time management skills so would be able to plan my week carefully to ensure I could do the appropriate PBL preparation whilst also attending lectures, dissection sessions and clinical skills sessions. I've demonstrated my time management skills already in my role as a prefect at school and by organising the publication of my school yearbook whilst also performing well in my school exams and working in a local care home in my spare time.

Secondly, I learn well by discussing new topics and ideas. This would mean I would actively participate in a PBL group and encourage others to do the same. I've demonstrated my communication skills by debating on the school debating team.

Thirdly, I am aware of my limits, and so would be very open about asking questions when I don't understand something. This is very important in PBL because it facilitates conversation and will ensure I cover issues in enough breadth to make me a safe clinician. I have demonstrated this by asking for help in my coursework at school when necessary."

Don't forget to finish well:
I believe these skills would help me function well in a PBL group.

Some positive attributes of PBL group members:
* Not afraid to ask questions
* Listen carefully to others' points of view
* Encourage quieter members to get involved
* Well-prepared
* Motivated
* Disciplined enough to study alone
* Pragmatic – you know what information would be important to know in a given situation

3.2   (T) What would you do if you couldn't ever study medicine?

This question aims to indirectly expose your inner disposition and determine your level of commitment. You should still provide an answer for the alternative career but its values should be congruent with the values of a doctor. If your reasons for studying medicine include altruism, scientific interest and working in a team, a possible different career path would be to become a Physician Associate. Physician Associates are a new and expanding profession in the NHS and their primary role is to support junior doctors. What is more, in using Physician Associates in your answer, you are also demonstrating an awareness of changes within the NHS.

Answer in three parts:

1. **Make it clear you are very committed to a career in medicine**
    "I am exceptionally committed to pursuing a career in medicine; however, if after numerous attempts I remained unsuccessful, I would still like to combine my passion for science, altruism and teamwork in another caring profession."

2. **Explain your alternative career plans**
    "I would consider becoming a Physician Associate. Physician Associates work with junior doctors, clerk patients, order tests and diagnose patients. They work in different specialties and have become an established member of the medical team. Their training involves learning core sciences and physical examination skills, both of which deeply interest me. As a Physician Associate, I would be able to apply my knowledge in challenging circumstances. Their work closely complements that of a junior doctor."

3. **Tell the interviewer why you are choosing medicine instead**
    "However, there are reasons why the role of Physician Associate is not my first career choice. The Physician Associate qualification currently allows for limited career progression. I really enjoy science, and medicine also offers a more rigorous training in science. I enjoy practical tasks and am quite dexterous, so I would like the opportunity to develop my practical skills and be able to perform a wider range of procedures. Medicine offers an opportunity to apply a combination of deep scientific knowledge and procedural skills to help people, which is why I want to become a doctor."

Other potential career choices:

*   Nursing
*   Medical relief worker
*   Basic sciences
*   Voluntary work
*   Allied healthcare professional

3.3 (T) Please give an example of when you demonstrated your effectiveness as a leader in a group situation.

This question is seeking an example. For any question that asks for an example, you can answer using the 'BARL' technique:

Background (i.e. set the scene)

Action (what YOU did to demonstrate the skill asked about in the question)

Result (what were the positive results of your actions?)

Link to medicine (why is the example relevant to your medicine application?)

Firstly, consider what the key qualities of a good leader are. A good leader is one who is fair, decisive, encouraging of the development of members in the group, diplomatic, organised, approachable and dependable. The example you choose should demonstrate some of these qualities. Think about the last time you had more input or decision-making responsibility than other team members in a group, whether in your part-time job, or during a school project. You must relate this to how the qualities you demonstrated in previous leadership roles have taught you how to be a good leader in future. This requires a degree of self-reflection: what did you do that worked well as a leader? Was there anything problematic that happened during your leadership, and if so, how did you resolve it? Being a good leader includes being able to keep those positive attributes in stressful situations.

A good example would be:

Background: *"I was a part-time salesperson at a vintage clothing shop, and had been working there for three years. On one of my Saturday shifts, the manager approached me, saying she had to leave immediately to deal with a family emergency. The manager asked me to tend to the shop and lead the rest of the team, consisting of four other workers. I had never done this before, and it was a particularly busy day for the shop but I agreed to do so. The pace in the shop quickly picked up and the workers were really stretched."*

Action: *"I strategically placed one worker at the door to greet customers, two on the sales floor and one by the cashier's till. I floated around the shop assisting the workers as much as possible. Later, I noticed a customer arguing with the worker who was on cashier duty. Seeing the look of panic on the cashier's face, I quickly went over and talked sensitively with the customer. The customer seemed reassured and happily made her purchase. At the end of the day, I played an equal part in cleaning up and ensured that everything was in order before closing the shop."*

Result: *"The other staff commented on how supportive I had been and how I had clearly given direction throughout the day."*

Link to medicine: *"I believe this ability to work alongside others will allow me to function well as a leader in a medical team."*

3.4 (T) What do you consider to be your weaknesses, and how might these affect your ability to perform in the role of a doctor?

It may seem counterintuitive to talk about your weaknesses in an interview, but it is the role of the interview panel to judge your suitability for their medical course and a future career in medicine. This can only be done effectively if your weaknesses, as well as your strengths, are properly explored.

Needless to say, if you are reluctant to work in a team or unwilling to deal with uncertainty and risks, this would not benefit your chances of successfully demonstrating your suitability for medicine. However, presenting one or two weaknesses that would not preclude you from a career in medicine, and using these effectively to show evidence of personal insight, self-reflection, and, most importantly, the initiative to take appropriate steps to deal with them, demonstrates that you possess what are highly sought-after qualities in medicine. On the other hand, if you were to say you had no weaknesses you would come across as either dishonest or someone who lacks insight.

The value of insight and reflective practice cannot be overstated. Working within the limits of one's competence is one of the duties of a doctor. Mindful of this, the following would be a suitable answer:
"I have very high expectations of myself, which means I can sometimes be quite self-critical if I make a mistake."

Now explain how this might affect your ability to perform in the role of a doctor, e.g.:
"If not dealt with appropriately, this might cause me to become easily frustrated with myself, which could add unnecessary stress to what is already a stressful job."

Finally, show that you have reflected on your weakness and taken the initiative to overcome it, e.g.:
"I have therefore taken the opportunity to reflect on this and realise that mistakes, especially within a safe learning environment, form an essential component of the learning process as they enable me to identify key areas that may require more practice, a different approach, or additional support."

The following is a good example for graduate applicants:
"I do not come from a science degree background, which means I may require more time to grasp some of the new concepts presented to me during the course. However, I have reflected on this and feel that my 'A' in A level Biology combined with 1st class honours in my Bachelors degree demonstrates that I have the ability to do well. Moreover, I have spoken with similar students at the medical school and feel that the combination of the excellent support they receive and my characteristic determination will enable me to excel."

3.5 *(MMI) You have just received your recent medical school exam grade, which you found disappointing. In fact you may have to repeat some modules. What would you do next to deal with this situation?*

Even the brightest student will not do well in medicine if they have poor coping strategies, and it is likely they will perform unexpectedly on at least one assessment during their time in medical school. It is important to remember that a career in medicine is a marathon, not a sprint, and there are a few things to keep in mind when answering this question. How have you dealt with poor results in the past? Perhaps on your mock A level or UKCAT exams? Alternatively, when have you been in a position where your expectations of yourself have not been met? Interviewers will be looking for the following:

- **Your ability to accurately reflect on the situation in which you have failed**

Reflection has become a very important part of the undergraduate and postgraduate medical curriculum, and in practice doctors are expected to appraise themselves critically. As such, routinely looking through your performance and assessing yourself is a good habit to form early in your medical career. Reflecting involves critically thinking about your development, what your learning needs are, and how you can meet them. A good medical student would reflect on why they think they performed poorly, how it makes them feel, and what they should be doing in order to do better on the next exam.

- **Your resilience in being able to put aside your disappointment in order to understand what went wrong**

Perhaps you would take a break by playing a game of rugby, or relaxing with a friend before returning to the situation and re-analysing it. It is important to mention this, as you cannot simply say you "wouldn't feel upset". This is a good opportunity to show your coping mechanisms and resilience.

- **What action you took to ensure success on your next attempt**

It is often difficult to look at a situation where you expected success, and understand what went wrong by yourself. In medical school you will likely have a lot of academic and pastoral support, and it is important to demonstrate a willingness to seek help when you have failed. This shows a genuine interest in improving and an understanding that sometimes you need someone else's perspective. Of course, after identifying areas for improvement you will need to define a clear plan such as: a revision timetable, scheduled extra tuition time, cutting back on extra-curricular activities temporarily, or even resitting some modules.

3.6 (T) Outside of the medical school curriculum and academic activities, how would you contribute to this university?

Universities may ask a question similar to this at the end of interview and the question may even be posed by a current medical student on the panel. The purpose of the question is to find out what type of person you are and whether you would fit into life at the medical school.

The question gives you an opportunity to briefly mention your extra-curricular achievements, whether that is music, sport or leadership. You also need to tie these into the opportunities available at the university. This is particularly important as it demonstrates that you have assessed whether the university is the right one for you.

Aside from your current interests, if you're able to find a new opportunity with a club or society that takes your liking, mention it! It gives you the chance to state why you think having interests outside of medicine is beneficial.

You could structure your answer into themes of extra-curricular activities, e.g.:
Music: *"For the last four years, I have been learning to play the piano and have worked hard to quickly attain a distinction in Grade 5. I've been able to join the school band and regularly play at school concerts. I hope during my time at medical school that I can join the Music Society and perform in their monthly concerts."*

Sport: *"I have played rugby since Year 7, representing my school every year, and this year I was selected for the 1st XV rugby team. I would really like to continue playing and would look forward to contributing to the medical school's rugby team, especially for the annual varsity match."*

Leadership: *"As my form representative, I spoke on behalf of my class in teacher–student feedback sessions. I was passionate about improving the teaching and extra-curricular activities within my school. I want to continue this by being a part of the student union, and if elected, to represent the views of my classmates to the faculty."*

Cultural: *"I've found that the university has an Afro-Caribbean/Indian/Iranian society, which is something I would really like to be a member of. I know they put on an annual student cultural show, which I would like to take part in."*

Something new: *"I've wanted to learn how to scuba-dive, and I know the dive club here offers lessons for an open water qualification. It would be great if I could join the club and take advantage of this."*

You can link what you say back to medicine:
"I would balance contributing to the extra-curricular activities at the university with achieving the best possible medical education. I've demonstrated my ability to manage my time by performing well in my GCSEs whilst also being orchestral lead at my school."

3.7 (T) Tell me about a time when you were criticised unfairly. What did you do?

During their professional career, everyone will receive criticism from colleagues. Whilst it is relatively obvious that the interviewers want to see how you react to criticism, the addition of 'unfairly' can be misleading and may tempt the interviewee to not admit they were in any way at fault, which you should avoid! Rather, a balanced answer where you reflect on the possibility that you were wrong will demonstrate to the examiners that you're able to critically appraise yourself. In addition, the interviewers are looking to see how you dealt with the situation, how you cleared the air and moved forward.

> **TOP TIP** Since this question is seeking an example, you should answer this question using the 'BARL' technique you learnt about in *Question 3.3*: **B**ackground, **A**ction, **R**esult and **L**ink to medicine.

Of importance here is the 'action' component. Some of the actions you might want to discuss are:

- **Recognise that you are not perfect**: Everyone makes mistakes, and when initially faced with a challenge to your work, have an open mind to recognise that perhaps you may have made a mistake.
- **Check your work**: State that if a potential mistake were identified, you would check that your work was accurate.
- **Take on board the criticism**: You don't necessarily have to agree with everything the other person says, but by listening to their point of view you demonstrate a desire to improve and that you are 'teachable'.
- **Clear the air**: This is a very important feature that most people forget to do, which can lead to increased tension within teams and an unfavourable working environment. If you did feel you were criticised particularly unfairly, this is the time to bring it up. Ask your colleague if you can have a word with them privately, and sensitively explain your thoughts.
- **Present a solution for the future**: This will prevent the same mistake happening again both from your side (if the mistake was yours) or from your colleague if they unfairly criticised you.

This structure represents an ideal way to react. If you didn't do one of these things in the example you give, don't worry – acknowledging that you are not perfect will show humility to the interviewer.

Similar rules to the *"Tell us about your weaknesses"* question apply here: don't feel pressured to come up with an original answer or a particularly difficult situation that you were put in. Certainly, don't exaggerate a simple situation or describe a mistake so terrible that it would make it difficult for the interviewers to grant you a place at medical school! Rather, an example that covers as many of the points above will score you more points, and make you look a better candidate in front of your interviewers.

3.8   (T) Where do you see yourself in ten years' time?

In ten years' time you will likely be in the middle of specialty training. Give an answer that shows you that you are a well-rounded, but fully committed individual.

Show that you have thought about your career and have used your past experience to explore what areas interest you. However, also demonstrate that you are aware that your medical experience is limited and that you are open-minded and keen to explore your options:
"In ten years' time I hope to be in the middle of specialist training. I have really enjoyed shadowing a cardiology consultant during work experience at my local hospital, and this is something that really interests me. However, I'm sure that I will find many other areas that interest me during my training and I am very keen to explore all the different options available."

Demonstrate skills that you have already gained, and how they will be useful as a doctor:
"Throughout my time at school I have developed many other skills, which I hope to continue to develop over the next ten years. For example, I have captained the hockey team for the past two years, which has taught me leadership skills and also how to adopt the role of a team player, helping everyone to achieve their full potential and work effectively as a team. I hope that in ten years' time I will be learning new management skills and working successfully in a multidisciplinary healthcare team."

Use examples to validate what you are saying and also show that you know what opportunities there are as a doctor, other than treating patients:
"I would also love to teach others during my career as a doctor, and in ten years' time I would like to be leading small group medical student teaching sessions. I have been tutoring three children at my local school, which has been very rewarding and something that I would like to continue with during university and as a doctor. This would allow me to build on my communication skills as well as helping others around me. Research is another exciting area that I haven't had much involvement in. I would like to use the upcoming years to get involved in some clinical research, and plan to make time in my future career to carry out research and audits to improve medical care."

Finish by showing that you have considered your work–life balance:
"I am a keen runner, and have been heavily involved in the athletics team at my local club and recently completed the London marathon. I hope that I will make the time around work to ensure that I still enjoy my hobbies, as this will keep me fit and allow me to maintain a good work–life balance when things get stressful. I am a very motivated individual and I'm sure I will do everything I can in the next ten years to ensure I am a successful and passionate doctor, while still enjoying a wide variety of extra accomplishments."

3.9   (T) Who has had the biggest positive influence on your life and why?

This question is about selecting what qualities you think are important in a person. It doesn't matter who the person you pick is, but why you pick them is important. You need to be careful that you don't spend your whole time talking about the person that influenced you, but rather about yourself and how this person had an impact on *you*.

Pick a variety of three or four key qualities that you can use to build your answer, such as:

- Hard-working
- Good listener
- Selfless
- Dedicated
- Empathetic
- Optimistic
- Competent
- Enthusiastic
- Honest

An example of a comprehensive answer would be:

*"Many people in my life have been very inspiring and have taught me which qualities I admire in a person. My aunt is someone who has had a major influence on my life and has really been an inspiration. She works as a primary school teacher, and is very **passionate** about her work. As well as working in a local hospital for a week, I did a week of work experience with her and saw how **dedicated** she was with the children; she was always **enthusiastic** and **optimistic**. Whenever there was a problem, she would always remain positive and use her skills and knowledge to overcome the problem and ensure the child was getting the best education possible. This is something that I would like to adapt to my career as a doctor. By using my calm attitude and positive approach I hope I will be as caring towards my patients as my aunt is towards her schoolchildren. My aunt is also a mother of two, and often looked after my brother and me. She always managed to balance her work and home life; even when things were stressful at work she wouldn't let that affect her when she came home and had to care for her children. I think this is a very important quality, especially as a doctor. Work can be stressful and time consuming but it is vital to have a good approach and remain positive to ensure you enjoy your career and home life."*

Remember it's quality and not quantity that is important. Don't just list ten traits that you think are important. Give a few traits and then back them up with examples and how they relate to a career in medicine. Try to show what traits you possess at the moment and how you would like to develop them further in your career.

3.10 (T) Why did you choose to apply to medicine as a postgraduate? What do you feel you have gained from your previous degree and how will it help you in medicine?

This is a bit of a sneaky question as it's three massive ones rolled into one. Try to split it into sections, ensuring you cover your motivation to study medicine, how your degree links to medicine and how this would help you be a better medical student.

They are trying to gauge what transferable skills you think you can apply from your previous studies. Try to think of general skills your degree has taught you, then expand on them and say why they would be useful in medicine.

Start by describing why you have chosen to apply to medicine now. This will vary from person to person but try to draw on the answer you had for 'why medicine?' Incorporate specific things such as interesting work experience, a placement you did during your degree or your final-year research project to show that your interest in the field was either deepened during your course or confirmed. The next important thing is to emphasise how much your previous degree makes you a better candidate for the course.

Next, try to give three or four skills you have gained, an example for each, and link them to how this would make you a better medical student. You could mention things like:

- **Independent study skills**: e.g. *organising information, managing your own time. Emphasise this if you are applying for a PBL course!*
- **Team working skills**: e.g. *a university group project you did – what did you learn from it?*
- **Ability to reflect, evaluate and analyse**: e.g. *did you learn to think critically during your final-year project?*
- **Being proactive or using your initiative**: e.g. *were you part of a society fundraiser? Were you involved in, or did you lead a project?*

A good example answer would be:
"I feel that I have gained many transferable skills that I can apply as a medical student. For example, I was really able to enhance my analytical and critical thinking skills through undertaking a research project where I conducted a literature review on chemical engineering. This has allowed me to learn about thinking logically and having attention to detail. These skills will be important as a medical student as I realise reflective learning is an important part of medicine and I will often have to reflect on my clinical skills and interaction with patients to inform my future practice."

3.11 (T) We see that you are a postgraduate. Tell us about your final-year research project – what did you gain from it?

Like the previous question, the main thing in this question is to emphasise which transferable skills you gained from your project and how this will help you as a medical student. You do not need to go into a lot of detail about the project; a short statement about the main idea of your project will be fine. Think back to your abstract and try to summarise it in two lines. Convey the main aim, the brief method and what you found. Even though you may have been working in a group, avoid the use of 'we' and instead use 'I' as much as you can to emphasise your role in the group and what you learnt.

You could begin with:
"My final-year project was a laboratory-based project regarding X; the main method was Y and the main findings were Z."

Next, you could mention some skills, giving examples for one or two of them and round off with how they would help you in medicine. Skills you could mention are:
- Problem solving – did your project go to plan? Did you have to troubleshoot any issues?
- Analytical/critical skills – what did you learn from doing the literature review?
- Practical skills – did you learn any specific technical skills to record data, such as PCR (polymerase chain reaction), thus demonstrating attention to detail?
- Presentation skills – did you have to produce a seminar or oral presentation outlining your work?

For example:
"I gained several transferable skills such as problem solving and having to think critically, as during the project I initially wasn't achieving results. I had to stand back and think about how I could adapt the method to produce results. This skill will equip me well as a medical student, as I realise I will often have to stand back and reflect about how I interact with patients and then adapt my practice to continually improve."

To end, you might want to briefly mention how you realise the importance of research in medicine and how your final-year project really emphasised this:
"Finally, the project emphasised to me the importance of research in medicine and how research can be applied in clinical practice, especially the 'bench to bedside' model. For example, I realise in medicine that an evidence-based approach is extremely important."

3.12 (T) You mention that you have experience of teaching – what have you learnt from this? Why are teaching skills important in medicine?

The main aims in answering this question are getting across that teaching is an important part of being a doctor and that you possess the relevant skills. Remember, for skills-based questions you may want to begin by using a broad opening statement:
"I realise that teaching is an important part of medicine and being a doctor."

You can then give examples of specific skills that you learnt as a teacher and by using a 'linking phrase', relate this to how it might be useful as a doctor or medical student. Avoid just listing skills, but instead try to use concrete examples to illustrate that you really understand that doctors are also teachers and how it is a key part of their role.

TOP TIP Don't forget to be logical in how you structure your answer if you are going to list multiple skills, e.g. *"Firstly,…Secondly,…Finally,…"*. This makes it much easier for the interviewer to follow your conversation.

For example: *"Firstly, by teaching first aid I understand that pupils have differing needs and that the work has to be adapted to their needs so that they can make progress. In the same way, I realise that as a doctor I will need to be aware that patients have differing needs or different levels of understanding of a condition or of a treatment. Therefore, this experience has taught me how to tailor my communication skills appropriately."*

Other skills that you may have learnt from teaching could be:
- **Communication**: Relaying complex information in an appropriate way by breaking it down into small chunks – doctors must teach patients in many ways, e.g. explaining about conditions, procedures, treatments. Patients often have different levels of understanding.
- **Reflective skills**: Evaluating my own performance regularly as a teacher as well as individual students' progress to inform future lessons. Reflecting is important as a doctor to inform future practice and in continuing professional development.
- **Leadership skills**: Through leading a class, motivating and engaging them. Often doctors have to teach other colleagues or students, either as a doctor on the wards or as an academic doctor in universities.

If you have time, for any of the above you can give a specific example using the '**BARL**' style of providing examples.

3.13 (T) What qualities do you possess that you think are necessary to make a good doctor?

This question is an opportunity for you to sell your own skills and experiences. The qualities that you possess will be personal to you.

Here are some ideas:
- People skills
- Leadership skills
- Teamworking skills
- Problem-solving skills
- Ability to cope under pressure
- Highly motivated and interested in their job and their patients
- Caring, compassionate and able to show empathy
- Trustworthy
- A strong desire to help others

Try to pick a few qualities that are different to each other but applicable to you. Give short examples to back these up.

> **TOP TIP** Each of these qualities could be used in a different style of question such as "Please give us an example of when you demonstrated your ability as a problem solver/team player/leader…." Ensure that you have thought about examples for each – perhaps by writing down occasions when you have demonstrated each of these. Why don't you do it now?
>
> **Example:**
> *"For me a good doctor is a strong communicator who works effectively as part of a team to make the right decisions for their patients whilst under pressure. They should also be compassionate, patient and able to empathise. Having completed my Duke of Edinburgh Gold Award I feel that I am good at working as part of a team to overcome challenges and find solutions to problems. I have also had experience of caring for others, having undertaken volunteer work at a care home. I helped the residents with eating their meals. I was surprised at how difficult this everyday task was for some [shows empathy] and I found it rewarding to help people with something so simple. Each of these skills will be valuable in a career as a doctor."*

3.14 (T) What does your best friend think about you applying for medicine?

Why am I being asked what my friend thinks about my career choice?

This sort of question may seem strange to you initially. It is simply another way of the interviewers asking you what qualities you have that make you suited to a career in medicine and that you have approached the career in a considered manner.

Think back to times when your friends have commented on you wanting to do medicine and what led them to make those comments:

If your best friend has specifically mentioned anything about you doing medicine, and it shows you in a good light, tell the interviewers! They might have seen you dealing with people in a very empathetic way and said you would make a great doctor. However, it is more than likely that your friends have not specifically made comments linking your good qualities to medicine, or anything about you doing medicine at all.

Link your qualities back to medicine and why they would be useful:

In this situation you can talk about other times people have picked up on the qualities that you think make you suited for medicine. Maybe your friends admire your strong work ethic and ability to do many extra-curricular activities without compromising on your studies, or they probably know how much you love science. Perhaps people come to you for advice as you are a good listener, and this could be another reason why you would make a great doctor.

Don't be embarrassed and just go for it!

People generally hate talking about their good qualities, which is why a question such as this makes it easier to do so. You can use actual experiences and compliments to your advantage, rather than being conscious of not coming across as arrogant.

> **TOP TIP** This question also gives you the opportunity to explain that you have discussed practicalities of a career in medicine with your friends.
>
> For example, you can mention that you discussed the challenges of the career (work–life balance, antisocial hours, long training pathways…) and the positives of the career (rewarding, interacting with people on a regular basis, intellectually stimulating…). You can mention how you come to medicine with a balanced, considered and mature viewpoint and discussing it with your friends has helped you come to this point.

3.15 (T) Please give me an example of how you have coped with failure.

Similar to previous questions about poor performance, criticism and weaknesses, you may feel you need to state that you have never failed or that if you admit to your failures, the interviewers will view this negatively. Remember that this is not the case! Irrespective of how successful or academically capable you are, you cannot have avoided failure through-out your entire life. Everyone has failures during their life and the interviewers know that you are not any different. Never say, *"I have never failed."* This is unlikely to be true, will come across as very arrogant and make the interviewers question your honesty.

Start the answer by first acknowledging the question:
"Even though I always try my very best in all my endeavours, I appreciate that failures are a natural part of life. I have failed many times in my life, but for each of my failures, I have made sure that I learn my lesson so that I don't repeat the same mistake."

This is a mature response. It shows that you are realistic and understand failures are inevi-table and that the most important thing is that you learn from them.

Next you need to back up your opening statement with a strong example (using the 'BARL' technique discussed in Question 3.3):
Background:
"For GCSE, I managed to attain 10A*s while playing football for my local club, practis-ing karate every week, and playing squash two or three times a week. I carried on with my busy sporting schedule during the start of my AS levels as I thought I would be able to juggle everything and also perform well in my studies. However, during a few class tests, I was getting very average and sometimes below average marks."

Action:
"I knew I had the potential to achieve better. I reflected and felt that the root cause was my extremely busy sporting schedule. Despite the fact that I loved all the sports I did, I knew I had to give some of them up to make sure I got the grades required to study medicine. I stopped playing squash and used that time to study harder."

Results:
"This had a dramatic effect and I managed to secure 3 As in my final AS level exams."

Link to medicine:
"From this experience I learnt a very important lesson on prioritisation. As a medical student I will need to decide when to cut back on some extra-curricular activities to ensure I meet my academic and clinical goals in medicine."

3.16 (T) We have thousands of medical applicants. Tell me something unique about you or something that you have done that sets you apart.

This is a question where you can really show off why you think you deserve a place over another applicant. Remember every student has good grades, sufficient work and voluntary experience. Think of something interesting and unique to you!

For example:
- Do you play a sport at a county/national level?
- Have you been on international expeditions e.g. World Challenge?
- Have you done a research project in the past?
- Have you set up a successful website?
- Do you have any non-traditional qualifications? e.g. qualified life guard or a qualified county cricket umpire

Begin by giving a summary of what you did. For example:
"From my background reading in biology I realised that there is an obesity epidemic happening, especially in Western societies, and this inspired me to undertake a small research project. I thought it would be interesting to assess the attitudes of my year group towards healthy living. I therefore designed a short questionnaire that assessed this and handed it out to my year group. I analysed the results and had very interesting findings."

Next explain what you learnt from doing this and link this into medicine.
For example:
"After analysing the results I was staggered to find that only 10% of my year exercised regularly. A good diet and physical exercise are essential components of a healthy lifestyle and it made me consider why the percentage was so low. I discussed these results with my head of year and proposed a plan on how to educate students at my school about healthy living. I believe a strong culture of healthy living needs to be built to fight off the rising obesity crisis."

This example answers the question that was asked, and also shows the interviewers that you are aware of important medical issues.

TOP TIP Always link your answer back to medicine and how the skills that you have acquired will help you become a better medical student and ultimately a better doctor:
"I believe it is particularly unique to have carried out a research project at this stage and I hope that it demonstrates that I have innovative academic skills which will stand me in good stead as a doctor."

3.17   (T) Tell me about your gap year and what you have learnt in the year out.

This is an open question and can be answered in a variety of ways. However, you can still use the opportunity to demonstrate that you are the ideal candidate for a position at medical school. Use this example framework:
*   Address why you took a gap year
*   What did you do for the year?
*   What have you learnt in the year?
*   How will the skills that you have learnt help you as a medical student and a future doctor?

For example:

"I took a gap year to have a year out from formal education and give myself time to travel, learn and explore. During my A levels, I spent a great deal of time and energy planning for the year ahead, which I believe greatly improved my time management skills. For example, to fund the year, I worked at a local shop at the weekends and some weekday evenings in the prior year. This meant I had to organise my study time very efficiently, which I believe will be an extremely useful skill at medical school."

In the above example, even before starting to talk about the gap year, the interviewer will be able to see important transferable skills were learnt (e.g. effective time management).
"I travelled to [insert country here] and volunteered at a rural hospital for a month. Here I had my first real insight into healthcare in a resource-poor country and a great appreciation of the healthcare we all take for granted back at home. I saw patients unable to afford to pay for an operation or the required medication. This had a deep impact on me and I started becoming interested in global health. I also interacted with many different people which I believe greatly enhanced my communication skills. Despite the extremely long hours in hospital, I thoroughly enjoyed it, which confirmed that medicine is definitely the career path for me."

Remember at the end of each section of your dialogue, reinforce what you have taken away and link it back to medicine.
*   Planning a gap year abroad – tell them how this involved a lot of organisation
*   Working part-time to fund your travels – developed time management skills
*   Meeting new people throughout your travels – improved your communication skills
*   Volunteering in a healthcare setting – reconfirmed your decision to study medicine

3.18   *How do you cope with stress? Give an example.*

This is a classic interview question that is applicable to any job or profession. It is commonly asked in medical interviews to help identify students who are able to cope with the challenges of being a doctor.

Recognising when you are stressed

It is important to explain how you recognise when you are stressed. Do you get grumpy? Does your heart rate rise or do you get sweaty? It is also important to say that you try to deal with the stress when you notice these things happening.

Seeking help

It is a good idea to mention that you would attempt to seek help from other people if it was due to a particularly difficult situation. Medicine is all about teamwork, and not attempting to handle things alone, e.g.:

"I tend to discuss the situation that made me stressed with my parents/friends; I find it useful to hear their thoughts and to look at the situation from different angles."

If it is a situation where your stress could result in harm to yourself or a patient it is important to say that you would immediately address the problem, e.g.:

"If I had too many jobs to do on the ward and trying to do them all myself would result in rash decision making, I would request help from other members of the team. I would step aside for five minutes to allow my mind to refocus before starting to work through the list of jobs again."

Now talk about anything you do to blow off steam; it's your opportunity to tell them a bit more about yourself

You can go on to talk about any extra–curricular activities you may do that help with stress, whether it be yoga or kick boxing. Perhaps you play a musical instrument or do oil painting and that helps with relaxation.

Choose an example (don't forget to use the 'BARL' technique that you learnt about in Question 3.3)

You can talk about any stressful situation you've come across, especially one that you think you dealt with well (and with the help of others). Make sure your answer lets you talk about a quality or skill that will be useful in medicine, and tie it in with a hypothetical scenario you may face as a doctor.

Chapter 4 | Hot topics in medicine

4.1   **(T) What do you think are the implications of surgeons having to report their outcomes?**

This question is testing whether you know about recent changes, which now make individual surgeons' results public – including their mortality (death) rates.

If you have been watching the news you will more than likely have heard about this.

The question is also testing whether you can explain why they should or should not be published. You should show understanding of both sides of the argument.

You can begin by explaining a short background to the question:
"Individual surgeons' data is now being reported publicly and compared to national averages. This has been heralded as a great innovation by some but criticised by others."

Now explain some of the pros and cons:
Pros of reporting:
- Makes the specialties more transparent.
- May highlight 'outliers' who are performing below standard, and make surgery safer.
- Helps patients to make an informed decision about who they would like to have operate on them.

Cons of reporting:
- May make surgeons 'risk averse', i.e. surgeons who used to operate on very complex and sick patients, some of whom may not survive, will stop operating on these cases (even though perhaps ultimately none would have survived without surgery). They may instead choose less complex cases only, because the high-risk patients make their figures look bad and may result in disciplinary action!
- May increase stress in what is already a very stressful profession.
- The outcomes are for individuals – not teams – but medicine is a team profession and the anaesthetists, physiotherapists, nurses and medical doctors will all care for the same surgical patient.

4.2 (T) What is your opinion on the NHS budget shifting from central control to the hands of Clinical Commissioning Groups?

This question is posed at two levels: the interviewer is assessing your awareness on a key change within the NHS whilst also assessing your ability to present a controversial issue. When discussing a controversial issue it is important to present a balanced argument. At the end, form your own opinion as required.

Familiarise yourself with the Department of Health White Paper: *Equity and Excellence* (2010):
www.gov.uk/government/uploads/system/uploads/attachment_data/file/213823/dh_117794.pdf

Commentary may be found on the health think tank King's Fund website:
www.kingsfund.org.uk/topics/nhs-reform/nhs-white-paper

You can begin by explaining the background:
"CCGs, Clinical Commissioning Groups, are regional groups of clinicians and lay advisors who decide which services to fund in their area."

Now explain some of the pros and cons:
Pros of CCGs:
- Empowers those who have direct patient contact to allocate funds for patient services in their area.
- CCGs incorporate primary care doctors, secondary care doctors and nurses, giving validity to the decisions CCGs make.

Cons of CCGs:
- Senior clinicians lose valuable clinical time to management. This is especially detrimental as there is a national shortage of doctors in some specialties.
- Clinicians have little formal training in financial management and are therefore relatively ill-equipped to manage a large sum of money.

Where you stand:
- I am cautiously optimistic about this change in management. I believe healthcare workers are best suited to advise how patient needs are best met. However, I do believe management training needs to be incorporated into medical education, so doctors have the right skills at their disposal.

4.3 (T) There has recently been a lot of news about the lack of GP trainees. What are your views on the current situation in general practice?

Besides providing evidence that you keep up-to-date with current affairs in medicine, this question also presents an opportunity to show that you can effectively communicate your views on complicated issues. You should begin with an opening statement to set the scene for your answer, e.g.:

"I feel that general practice is a fundamental part of the NHS, because it deals with 90% of NHS patient interactions, provides local healthcare in the community, and acts as a gatekeeper to hospital services."

Now introduce the issue at the centre of the current recruitment crisis:

"However, it has been reported that fewer than 25% of foundation doctors in 2014 intended to go into GP training, which is causing concerns over the recruitment of new GPs."

The interview panel is unlikely to ask you about specific figures. However, if you do happen to recall some statistics, you may include these to show that you have genuinely followed the topic. Be careful not to sound over-rehearsed, as an answer that is conveyed naturally usually makes a better impression.

Now give your views on this issue. You may want to start by suggesting what could be contributing to the recruitment crisis in general practice:

"I think there has been a change in the general perception of a GP career amongst medical students and junior doctors. This may be due to a combination of the growing demand for GP services, rising patient expectations and disproportionate funding. These may discourage medical students and junior doctors from choosing a career as a GP."

Try to conclude your answer by suggesting possible ways to deal with these conceptions:

"I feel it is essential for the Government to provide further funding for general practice so that GPs have the workforce capacity to properly deal with the growing demand and to provide a better service for patients. This could boost morale within general practice and demonstrate that the Government is supporting GPs."

TOP TIP Begin to foster an interest in current affairs in medicine. It is always much easier to answer a question when you have a genuine understanding of the topic.

4.4 (T) Please outline what you understand by the term 'three-parent babies' and describe the ethical concerns associated with the concept.

Whilst this is a challenging question it is assessing whether you keep up-to-date with current research topics in the news. A recent news item has been the House of Lords' approval of IVF-based fertility treatments in order to prevent 'mitochondrial disease'.

> **TOP TIP** A good way of keeping up-to-date is to read the major health news headlines from up to a year before your interview date.

To answer this question you need to be able to explain the basic principles behind three-parent babies. (If the interviewers are less harsh they may even provide a definition of the term for you. However, you will still need to be able to reference why it is such a hot topic in medicine, and as highlighted by the question, the ethical concerns.)

To begin you may choose to summarise the process:
"Three-parent babies are babies born as a result of a specialised in vitro *fertilisation process where the future baby's mitochondria come from a donor, meaning that the baby will have three different genetic parents."*

You can then explain why this may be done:
"The mitochondria are passed on exclusively from the mother; if the mother has a genetic mutation in her mitochondrial DNA she will pass it on to her child. This could lead to severe, life-limiting diseases, including muscular dystrophies and diabetes mellitus. Therefore if the mother's mitochondria are replaced with those from a healthy donor, these diseases may be prevented."

Finally you could discuss some of the ethical concerns such as:
* A child's sense of identity may be affected. If they are aware that they have three genetic parents, they may consider themselves to be different from other healthy children who have two parents.
* The long-term effects and safety of mitochondrial DNA replacement are still largely unknown. It may have implications later in life.
* Critics may argue that scientists are 'playing God' and just because this can be done, does not mean that it should be done.
* There is research to suggest that the majority of mitochondrial diseases are caused by mutations in the nuclear DNA that encodes for elements of the mitochondria. Therefore replacing mitochondrial DNA may not prevent the disease at all.

4.5 (T) Genetics is having an increasing importance in medicine. Why is this? What role can you see it having in the future of medicine?

Whilst this may seem to be a very wide question, you can concentrate on some key ways it may affect clinical medicine.

You can mention that you are aware of various ways that genetics can impact medicine or is a growing research area and that it has many ethical implications. You might want to mention a news item that you have recently seen. You could mention:

- Current genetic research helps us find out more about certain diseases and the genetic basis of them, which may help in **more effective management**, e.g. diseases such as diabetes or mental health disorders such as schizophrenia.
- Some genetic variations (and as such the diseases which they lead to) are inherited. Genetic research helps us to understand **disease susceptibility** in families and ethnic groups who possess these variations.
- Genetic research may inform **drug development** by defining new drug targets.
- Genetic research may enable the development of **personalised medicine**, i.e. drugs that are tailored to our genetic profiles so that they have fewer side–effects for each individual.
- Increased **accessibility of 'genetic sequencing' (i.e. 'genetic testing')** means that we can now screen for certain genetic disorders.

If you have time, you might want to mention 'epigenetics' (the concept that some chemicals can turn certain genes on or off), which is a current hot topic in genetics – you may want to read more about this online.

If you can think of an example to illustrate each point, it will really show your interest and also that you keep abreast of medical news. To conclude you may want to briefly mention the ethical concerns of genetic medicine:

"Though there are numerous ways that genetics can impact the future of medicine, I am aware that there are several ethical considerations such as...:"

- What should we permit genes to be used for?
- How should we gain access to genes? (should they be just from consenting adults?)
- How do we ensure confidentiality of the stored genetic material and the data we gain from it?

4.6   (T) What are the consequences of obesity for health services? Why?

This question is testing your knowledge on the current obesity epidemic, the reasons behind it and the impact on the NHS of the increasing number of obese patients.

You can start by giving some of the consequences of obesity (BMI ≥ 30kg/m²) on the individual, as this in turn will impact how they use healthcare services:

*   Joint pain
*   Mobility issues
*   Increased risk of cardiovascular disease (strokes and heart attacks)
*   Increased risk of type 2 diabetes.

Now you can explain how these problems in each individual go on to affect the NHS:
"These conditions are seen more frequently due to the increasing number of obese patients in the population. This can lead to...:"

*   More visits to the GP, A&E and hospital referrals
*   An increase in certain procedures, e.g. joint replacement surgery and bariatric surgery
*   Increased prescription of medication to control high blood pressure, high cholesterol and diabetes
*   An increase in community care after strokes and for those with decreased mobility
*   Patients with multiple conditions and therefore complex (and expensive) healthcare issues.

As a final part to this question you can then go on to describe the impact of an increase in obesity on the healthcare system as a whole:

*   In a 'limited pot' of funding, when more resources are directed towards obesity, it may result in less money being directed towards other healthcare areas, e.g. cancer therapies.
*   Obese patients are often more complex to treat in hospitals – they are higher risk surgical candidates and they require special 'bariatric' equipment. This not only poses extra risks to the patient but makes care more challenging.

4.7 *(MMI) You are working for the NHS organ donation programme. Wales has recently introduced a 'soft opt-out' system for organ donation. You are asked to explain to a patients and relatives group what is meant by the 'opt-in' and 'opt-out' systems. Explain some of the pros and cons of each to the group. You have 7 minutes. Your interviewers (x2) will play the role of patients/relatives.*

This question is testing your knowledge of organ donation systems. It is also assessing your ability to convey the information using minimal jargon. This topic has received regular media coverage, particularly as Wales became the first part of the UK to change to an opt-out system in December 2015. You need to be familiar with the current opt-in donation system in the rest of the UK and the arguments for introducing an opt-out system.

Organ donation can be an emotive subject so you will need to convey your opinion sensitively.

Start by introducing yourself, and finding out what the patients/relatives know already: *"Hello, my name is Tim. I work for NHS Blood and Transplant and I have been asked to discuss organ donation. Can I ask what you know about the current system in Wales and if you are aware of any changes that are going to be made?"*

Listen to the patients' responses and then give some background to organ donation in the UK: *"Currently, UK residents can register to donate all or some of their organs for transplant after their death. This is called an opt-in system. In an opt-out system it is presumed that every individual consents to donating their organs after their death unless they actively declare that they do not wish to donate. Under a soft opt-out system (such as the new Welsh system) families will still be consulted to make the final decision."*

Arguments for changing to an opt-out system:
- Many people who wish to donate 'haven't got round' to signing the register. Making this easier will increase donations.
- It reduces pressure on relatives at the time of death as their loved one could have opted out if they strongly objected to donation.
- Many families decline to donate their relatives' organs, as they don't know what the deceased would have wanted.

Arguments for keeping the current opt-in system:
- The shift from 'giving' to 'taking' organs may be seen negatively and the public may perceive the state to be 'snatching' organs.
- Donation should remain voluntary.
- Concerns over the ease of opting-out. Vulnerable people or those not 'in the know' may not opt out even though they object to donation.
- Preference for alternative programmes to recruit more donors.

4.8   (T) What are your views on using alternative medicine, such as homeopathy, as a form of treatment?

This question tests your background knowledge on medical issues. To approach this question you need to have a basic understanding of what alternative medicine and homeopathy are.

Begin by explaining or defining what these terms mean.

Remember the interviewers are not looking for you to recite a memorised phrase that you obtained from a website. This will make you look as if you don't understand the topic in question.

"Alternative medicine is a form of treatment that falls outside mainstream healthcare. Homeopathy is a form of alternative medicine. In homeopathic treatments, it is believed that diluting the drug or substance in water increases its concentration because the water is supposed to have a form of 'memory'."

Remember there is a difference between 'alternative medicine' and 'complementary medicine'. Make sure you know and understand the difference. Next explain what your views are.

TOP TIP Your interviewers are clinicians and scientists. The practice of Western medicine is evidence-based. This means that decisions such as what treatment to give, when to give it, and for how long are determined by evidence from scientific studies. For the vast majority of alternative medicine there is little scientific evidence to show that it is effective. Whilst there are arguments in favour of alternative medicine, if your views are pro alternative medicine (especially pro homeopathy), it may be wise not to publicise this too loudly at the interview.

After explaining what alternative medicine and homeopathy are, you should give a balanced but cautious summary of the therapy, e.g.:

- Give a brief overview of the different types of alternative medicines you know.
- Explain why it is not used routinely in healthcare.
- Distinguish 'alternative medicine' from 'complementary medicine' – there are lots of definitions available online.
- Explain the basics behind homeopathy.
- Explain the negatives of homeopathy (lack of evidence for its efficacy) but balance this with arguments about why it has been funded on the NHS previously (e.g. some argue that in certain individuals it can reduce use of acute hospital beds for chronic symptoms, saving the NHS money).
- Explain that your views on homeopathy are purely evidence-based and you would advocate its use in the future only if substantial evidence becomes available showing its efficacy. As a doctor you will often completely change your practice as new evidence emerges.

4.9   (T) Do you think a 24/7 GP service is a move in the right direction for the NHS?

There is no 'right' answer to questions such as this. Questions with a political dimension can bring a real spectrum of opinion, often with some people feeling particularly strongly one way or another. As such this is an ideal opportunity to not only communicate your own opinion, but also to demonstrate that you are open-minded, sensitive and respectful of others' beliefs.

"Whilst the details of this plan are evolving, the main thrust of the plan is to increase access to all healthcare services, particularly general practice, and to try to standardise the quality of care across the entire week."

Of course it is a noble idea to try to improve ease of access to healthcare – most interviewers are not particularly interested in you emphasising this and would far rather you spend your time addressing the practicalities of how this would work in the real world of financial constraints and the limitations of other resources such as trained staff.

It would be interesting to discuss which sections of society may be most in need of increased opening hours. You could demonstrate your knowledge of the health service by pointing out that access to GPs is very variable across the country, and that some practices already open at weekends and offer extended opening during the working week.

It is worth extending the scope of the question to add some context – quality of care in hospitals is reported to be different at weekends. Whilst this quality of care has not been linked exclusively to staffing there are usually only emergency staff in each specialty in the hospital at weekends. There are moves afoot to alter the historical staffing patterns in secondary care, bringing more senior staff into the hospital in what were previously considered 'out-of-hours' periods.

Whilst it is advisable to have a 'balanced viewpoint' as demonstrated above, you may be pushed to give an answer. Be prepared for this. You can summarise your thoughts in a sentence such as:
"Whilst there are noble intents by asking GPs to work a 24/7 service, there are also considerable challenges such as the need for a larger GP workforce and more NHS funding (which may divert funds from other sectors, e.g. cancer therapy). At a time when the NHS is attempting to make savings I don't feel that a 24/7 GP service should be the priority."

4.10 *(MMI) It has been suggested that pharmacists and nurses should be given more responsibility, such as prescribing, to relieve demands on the health service. Please discuss with the interviewer the advantages and disadvantages of giving other healthcare professionals more responsibility to prescribe medications. You have 7 minutes.*

This question will test your reasoning skills as well as draw on your knowledge of the current workings of the NHS.

Healthcare workers (other than doctors) have been able to prescribe for a long time in the NHS. Midwives frequently prescribe drugs involved in pregnancy and senior nurses who have completed a prescribing course also have the ability to prescribe. It is also important to note that prescribing limitations are often imposed to match an individual's role and level of training (e.g. a junior doctor may not be able to prescribe some chemotherapy drugs). These are essential to ensure individuals do not prescribe beyond their competence. Prescribing is likely to be the most potentially harmful responsibility you have as a junior doctor.

Don't portray doctors as omniscient pharmacologists or downplay other healthcare workers such as nurses, many of whom have a wealth of knowledge and experience. It is true that medical training is longer and has a greater focus on understanding the physiology and pharmacology behind medications but that does not mean every doctor will know everything about every drug. Nurses are very practically trained and through experience will also learn to recognise when certain drugs are used.

Advantages
- Certain drugs are simple and safe to prescribe without extensive pharmacology knowledge.
- Nurses often spend more time with the patient and therefore may be better placed to decide when certain drugs are needed.
- It may reduce delays to drug prescriptions, especially at times when drugs are needed (e.g. pain relief) and other staff are very busy.
- It allows doctors more time for other tasks and may prevent rushed prescriptions.

Disadvantages
- Even the safest drugs can have 'contraindications' (i.e. reasons why they may not be safe to prescribe).
- A comprehensive understanding of pharmacology and physiology may be needed to avoid drug interactions and adverse reactions.
- It may confuse the issue of who has ultimate responsibility for patient care if other healthcare professionals can make independent decisions.

Once you have presented your balanced argument, try to conclude with a considered viewpoint, e.g. *"In conclusion, I think the expansion of prescribing power has many potential benefits, provided adequate training is given and appropriate boundaries are set."*

4.11   *(MMI) You are talking with a friend about 'whistleblowing'. Please explain to them what you understand by the term, whether you think staff should be encouraged to 'whistleblow' and what the potential challenges are. You have 7 minutes.*

Whistleblowing means reporting suspected wrongdoings, at an individual or organisational level, that may put patient safety at risk. The General Medicine Council advocates a culture where concerns should be raised about misconduct which may lead to harm, in order to protect patients and colleagues. Several cases exist where staff have allegedly experienced severe repercussions for raising concerns about wrongdoings, such as medical errors or poor management. Examples of high-profile cases include:

- High mortality rates of babies undergoing heart surgery at Bristol Royal Infirmary
- Organ retention without consent at Alder Hey Children's Hospital
- Failures of patient care at Mid Staffordshire NHS Foundation Trust
- Unsafe practice at a clinic where Baby P was seen before his death.

Then explain the challenges faced by those wishing to raise concerns:
Staff may not report concerns due to fear of retaliation or a lack of faith in the system. They may find themselves being victimised, intimidated and bullied. This culture of fear and silencing is not unfounded. In fact, a review carried out by a senior barrister, into failures at one NHS Foundation Trust, reported:

- 'Shocking' accounts of serious concerns regarding patient safety being rejected
- Disciplinary action taken against those who spoke out, frequently resulting in loss of jobs and serious psychological damage
- Staff being bullied and oppressed when attempting to speak up
- Significant deterrents and vindictive treatment of those raising the concerns, including bullying, harassment, replacement of supportive staff, deliberate increase in workload, counter-allegations and disciplinary action.

Now talk about what is being done to tackle this:
Legislation was recommended to protect whistleblowers from discrimination when seeking new employment, as well as the appointment of a national officer for whistleblowing and a whistleblowing guardian at every NHS organisation. The action plan also included many other measures to ensure concerns are investigated properly. Whether this will result in change of attitudes remains to be seen.

Finally give a balanced conclusion:
Whistleblowers have measurably increased the quality of care that patients receive over the years, but often at a great cost to themselves at a professional and personal level. Thus, changes need to be made to create a climate of openness in the NHS so that staff can raise legitimate concerns without fear of reprisal.

4.12 (MMI) You are an editor of a medical journal. You are asked to discuss with two co-editors about whether your journal should publish research funded by the drug industry. Two interviewers will play your co-editors. You have 7 minutes to discuss the issue with them.

The question is asking you to discuss the ethics of research funded by the drug industry. You may have a strong opinion, but it is crucial to provide arguments for both sides of the argument and conclude logically.

Start by giving an overview of the topic:
High-quality and non-biased information is needed to inform evidence-based medicine. The drug industry has a vested interest in having favourable research published; however, it also provides invaluable innovation and funds important research.

Arguments in favour of research funded by the drug industry:
- Competition in the industry drives innovation.
- Industry can provide a magnitude of funds to study and test multiple potential drugs for efficacy simultaneously, as well as gathering information about side-effects.
- Major breakthroughs made by the industry greatly benefit patients.
- Surgical innovation in collaboration with the industry provides new and innovative devices.
- Without the research funded by drug industry, there would be a much smaller pool of study results to draw on.
- Studies are still conducted in accordance with strict ethical guidelines.

Arguments against research funded by the drug industry:
- Questionable ability to act without bias.
- Vested interest in promoting company's products to increase market share.
- The risk that research outcomes may be promotional rather than educational.
- The risk that industry may only publish results that are in favour of the company interests and withhold unfavourable trial information.
- Drug development may not represent global burden of disease; instead funding may be directed towards research that is likely to be profitable.

Discussion
You could suggest some changes on behalf of the journal and its authors to maintain transparency:
- Monitoring by publicly funded organisations to help reduce bias.
- Research funded by industry should be accompanied by a commentary from independent reviewers in the same field.
- Ensure that clinician researchers operate independently in trials.
- Include teaching on the ethics of industry-funded research in medical school and postgraduate curricula for health professionals.

4.13 (MMI) You are talking with an IT developer. Have a conversation with her about how can we integrate the use of the internet and digital technology into the world of medicine. You have 7 minutes.

This question is not only a chance for you to show how much you know about technological advances in the field, but also gives you the opportunity to demonstrate your creativity and practical ideas.

The internet and digital technology are, of course, already somewhat integrated into our healthcare system. As well as using the internet to broaden our own knowledge as health professionals, there are tools such as 'NHS Choices' and digital health records that are already widely used; it would therefore be a good idea to begin by acknowledging the use of these in the field:

"The internet and the digital world are already important tools in medicine – for example…"

Once you have shown your awareness of what is already out there, the interviewers are interested in what extra ideas you have to offer. Use your own interests and experiences of the medical field to expand on existing ideas or come up with entirely new (and at least somewhat sensible!) ways of digitalising medicine. This is an example of a good elaboration:

"Speaking from personal experience, GPs seem to be a very digitalised specialty in medicine. Many GPs already use alternative methods of appointments, such as phone calls, video calls and even Skype appointments. In the coming years, this patient–doctor relationship could be even further digitalised, for example, by using entirely web-based consultations for the majority of patients with minor ailments. This might allow the doctors to spend valuable, extra time with more ill patients, such as those at the end of their lives."

It is also a good idea to keep an eye on the news for the latest technological developments in medicine. There will always be something new being introduced or trialled in hospitals, so you could perhaps talk about their implementation and how realistic/practical their use might be.

"Recently, in the news, I have heard about the introduction of an ultrasound app for all doctors in a hospital in X. The free app contains novel software to be downloaded onto the staff smartphones and it means that all doctors in this hospital essentially have a portable ultrasound with them at all times. As well as being an innovative idea, I think that it could really transform patient care and may even help reduce the duration of patients' stay in hospital."

4.14   *(MMI) You are speaking to an American friend, who tells you he has heard that the NHS chooses medicines based on their cost rather than their efficacy. Please discuss with him about the system for selecting medicines within the NHS. You have 7 minutes.*

This task has several elements to it. It tests your knowledge of the basics of resource allocation within the NHS and of the role of evidence-based medicine. Implicit in your friend's analysis is the suggestion that the NHS gives consideration *only* to the cost of treatments, rather than weighing up both the costs and benefits, when making a decision.

> **TOP TIP**   As this is an 'explaining' station, you should do all the things you would normally do when explaining a complex topic to someone. You should assess their knowledge of the subject first, giving information in small chunks and checking their understanding throughout.

"That is an interesting topic. The NHS hospitals actually do not choose medicines for themselves; rather, the NHS uses an independent organisation, NICE (The National Institute for Health and Care Excellence) to make recommendations on which treatments should be made available for use. NICE considers the evidence for each treatment before reaching a decision."

You should be aware of the work of NICE, and how the NHS uses the information generated by NICE to inform treatment selection.

"For each new treatment, a panel at NICE will consider not just the effectiveness of a drug in terms of its capacity to cure disease or extend life, but also the impact of its use on quality of life. The panel is made up of health professionals, academics and researchers, and may also include lay members, patients or patient advocates."

When discussing the aspect of cost, stay calm and resist taking a polemical standpoint. There is an element of truth to his statement – treatment costs *are* considered as part of the decision making process – so it won't do to reject his viewpoint completely.

It is fair to say that costs are considered by NICE as part of its assessment of the new treatment. However, this is just one aspect of the decision making process. A treatment with a strong evidence base (to improve not only quality but length of life, which is measured in a specific way called 'QALY' or 'Quality-Adjusted Life Years' – worth looking up on the internet!) is more likely to persuade the panel than one that is simply cheap.

End your explanation by checking to see if your friend is satisfied with the answer you have given, or if he has any residual questions.

Chapter 5 | Academic questions

5.1   (T) *What is the role of doctors in academia?*

Not all students will be interested in a career in academic medicine, but it is important to know the vital impact that academic clinicians have and the role they play in advancing the healthcare profession. If you are unsure whether you would prefer to be primarily a clinician versus an academic, feel free to say so! Medical school is a long period of time, and so is the period of training afterwards, so the interviewers aren't specifically looking for a personal answer to this question. You will have a lot of time to decide what direction you want your future career to take.

Academic clinicians may take on several roles as well as their clinical duties:

• **Researcher/scholar**

Students can choose to do intercalated degrees at medical school, and trainees can complete higher postgraduate degrees, such as Masters or PhD degrees. Doctors can be involved in clinical, translational or pre-clinical research. Clinical research involves the evaluation of changes in clinical practice. Translational research involves beginning to apply new basic science discoveries into clinical techniques or treatments, and evaluating their safety, efficacy and cost-efficiency, along with other parameters. Pre-clinical research involves the process of discovering something new that contributes to our understanding of a disease or its treatment, and often involves lab work. Each of these types of research allows medicine to progress. In your answer, try not to spend too much time defining these, but rather mention how research contributes to improving patients' lives.

• **Educator**

Many doctors are involved in the development and delivery of undergraduate and postgraduate medical curricula. Many will work for the university for a proportion of their week and will lecture as well as plan and deliver smaller group teaching sessions. They may also examine for the university or for a postgraduate body such as one of the Royal Colleges.

• **Leader/university administration**

Doctors are important stakeholders in the development of the healthcare system in which they work. Many doctors are involved in initiatives such as the Faculty of Medical Leadership and Management, help shape NHS policy and decide how healthcare in the UK is delivered. Without the expert advice from people at the frontline of patient care, the NHS would lack guidance, so it is important that you highlight this.

5.2   (T) Is medical research important and if so, why? Should all doctors be required to contribute academically to their field?

This is a question of two parts. For the first part of the question, you should:

- **Define what medical research is.** Read around the different types of research (as mentioned in the previous question) and study designs (*buzzwords to search on the internet are: prospective study, retrospective study, randomised control trial, case–control study, cohort study*) and the difference between audit (a method of ensuring we are performing at the required standard) and research (aims to answer a new question). If you can incorporate this into your answer, the interviewers will be <u>very</u> impressed.

- **Explain why medical research is important.** Research is what drives medicine forward. Without it, we would still be stuck in the Dark Ages. It is basically a laboratory experiment or a clinical study (which involves patients) and tests a hypothesis. The results are obtained and analysed and conclusions are made. Remember the practice of medicine is **evidence-based**! This means that clinical guidelines take into account evidence (experiments and clinical studies) that have been published in scientific papers.

Should all doctors be required to contribute academically to their field?

Remember 'academically' does not just mean doing research and writing papers. Read the previous question for other ways doctors can contribute academically. Contributing academically has both pros and cons and you should address both:

Pros:

- Doing research will add to the evidence base and ultimately aid in a better understanding of medicine and increased patient care.
- Teaching is crucial since healthcare in the future depends on competent effective doctors.
- By taking part in research, doctors can read other research with more understanding, and spot potential flaws in studies.

Cons:

- Doctors may not enjoy doing research. Mandating all doctors to perform research may result in poor quality research being performed.
- If the academic time comes out of time on their clinical day job this will decrease patient contact time.
- If all doctors have paid academic time in addition to patient contact time, we may not be able to sustainably fund the NHS.

5.3   (T) At what stage in one's medical career does learning stop?

The short answer to this question is never! However, expanding on this answer will allow you to impress your interviewers in a number of different ways: it will allow you to demonstrate a commitment to lifelong learning and to show off your knowledge regarding medical careers. Finally, you can use a relevant, specific example to highlight the importance of lifelong learning.

It would be a good idea to begin your answer with a strong statement that shows you appreciate that all doctors, even the most experienced consultants, never stop learning.

"I know that if I am granted a place to study medicine, my learning will not stop once I graduate from university; I intend to continue learning and updating my knowledge throughout my career."

Following this strong opening, you can then go on to elaborate, to turn a passable answer into a superb answer.

"I am aware that doctors, including consultants, attend conference and courses regularly to ensure that their professional knowledge is kept up-to-date. The GMC [General Medical Council: the body that regulates doctors] has recently introduced a process called revalidation, whereby doctors must formally demonstrate every five years that they are keeping their knowledge up-to-date in order to continue practising. If I work as a doctor, I will make the care of my patients my first concern, and I know that keeping my professional knowledge up-to-date is a key part of that."

This answer shows awareness of the working life of a consultant, and of the recently introduced GMC revalidation programme. To really stand out from the crowd you could even give an example of how important it is to keep up-to-date with medical knowledge:
"As an example of just how important lifelong learning and keeping up-to-date is, I know that in the 1970s, the idea that stomach ulcers were caused by bacteria was laughable – but that in 2005, two Australian researchers were awarded the Nobel Prize for Medicine after demonstrating exactly that!"

5.4 (MMI) This is a model of the DNA double helix. What relevance does this have to modern-day medicine? You will be shown a model of a double helix. You have 7 minutes to answer the question.

When approaching this question, it is important to ensure you actually discuss the question being asked; do not simply state facts you know about DNA (that isn't the question and the interviewers won't be expecting you to be a professor of genetic medicine!), but instead discuss the impact that DNA and its structure have in modern-day medicine.

TOP TIP Do not be thrown by the fact there is a DNA model in front of you. This question is similar to *Question 4.5* but asked in a more interactive/MMI format.

Broadly, there is no real right or wrong answer here; demonstrating a good knowledge of the area you choose to discuss and being ready to start a discussion with the interviewer on your choice of topic will form a strong base for any answer.

There are many areas in which DNA and genetics still influence modern-day medicine and a wide array of topics that could be chosen to answer this question, including:
- **Genetically modified bacteria in the production of insulin:**
  - Historically, insulin was only available by harvesting it from the pancreas of a pig, an expensive and labour-intensive process with added complications of potential allergic reactions
  - Nowadays, production of insulin from genetically modified bacteria allows diabetic patients access to cheap and widely available insulin without the additional risks of porcine insulin.

- **Greater understanding of how genes influence disease processes, allowing for genetic counselling and targeted treatments towards at-risk patient groups:**
  - For example, women with specific genes, but without symptoms, may choose to have a double mastectomy (removal of the breast tissue) 'prophylactically' (i.e. pre-emptively) due to an increased risk of developing the cancer in the future.

- **The ongoing research into treatments for genetically inherited conditions, such as sickle cell disease (SCD) and cystic fibrosis (CF):**
  - A relatively recent advancement is gene therapy, which replaces the faulty genes that are present in patients with these conditions and which may hold the future potential of cures for these genetic diseases.

As alluded to earlier, it is important to discuss any points you raise with the interviewer. Your interviewer may intentionally disagree with some of the points you raise. Do not be put off by this, as they will want to see you develop your answers and see how you think on your feet.

5.5 *(T) What is evidence-based medicine?*

This question is assessing what you know about evidence-based medicine and why it is important.

Start by defining what evidence-based medicine is, for example:
"Evidence-based medicine is the use of scientific research and clinical studies to inform decision making in patient care."

You can then go on by explaining how the 'evidence base' is formed:
"There are different types of studies that provide different levels of evidence:
- *'Systematic reviews' or 'meta-analyses' (studies which summarise all the research performed in a treatment area) are regarded as the best to use in decision making*
- *A 'randomised control trial' objectively compares one treatment with another and then, using statistics, can state the better treatment for patient outcome.*

Doctors can then use this information alongside their own judgment when treating patients."

You can then mention why evidence-based medicine is important:
- It improves patient outcomes. Basing decisions on studies removes the 'guesswork' from medicine. It means that every patient gets the best treatment possible, as demonstrated by science.
- It creates a healthcare system where treatment should be fair – patients with the same disease will be treated with the best treatment, regardless of which doctor they have. NICE produces guidelines based on evidence-based medicine that doctors should follow in day-to-day practice.
- It controls the treatments that are introduced to patients – all new treatments must be deemed to be safe and shown to be better or equivalent to the current treatment.

5.6 *(MMI) What is consent and for what reasons might someone lose their ability to consent to treatment? List as many as you can, and explain why they can't consent in each. You have 5 minutes.*

You may not know the legal guidelines for judging whether some has the ability (also known as 'capacity') to consent but you can work it out from first principles. Break down the question into its constituent parts. Explain what you understand by 'consent':

"Before a patient undergoes an examination, investigation, procedure or commences a treatment, their consent must first be obtained. This is the process by which their permission to proceed with the intervention is sought and gained."

Give more detail, ensuring you highlight your understanding of the role of the doctor or healthcare professional in this process.

"It is the responsibility of the healthcare professional to ensure the patient is fully informed as to the content of the intervention, its aims, risks and benefits, before making their decision. Their consent, if obtained, should be properly documented."

There are some specific qualities the patient should possess if their consent is to be considered truly informed.

"Under ideal circumstances, the patient should be able to understand the information given to them, retain that information long enough to come to a decision, and be able to communicate that decision. However, a deficit in any of these qualities, whether permanent or temporary, may affect their capacity to give informed consent."

Using this information, systematically list as many situations as you can, in which this capacity could be hindered. For example:

"A patient with dementia or learning difficulties may not be able to understand the information given to them. Likewise, someone who is seriously ill and losing consciousness, or is severely intoxicated, may be unable to reach any decisions about their own treatment. This also goes for those suffering acutely from psychiatric disorders such as schizophrenia, or certain forms of brain injury."

Don't forget that communication is essential for consent as well – there may be some unique situations where it is not possible to communicate with people, e.g. in an emergency scenario where a patient speaks a language for which there is no interpreter available (either in person or over the phone).

It's worth mentioning that capacity should be reassessed periodically, and that it should be assumed a patient is able to make his or her own decisions unless it can be demonstrated otherwise. You should also understand (broadly) how people who lack capacity are managed in the NHS.

5.7 (MMI) Medicine is constantly making advances in both the scientific and clinical fields. What do you think is the most important medical advancement in the past 200 years and why? You have 7 minutes to respond.

This question is a great opportunity for any interviewee to show an ability to form a well-rounded discussion. If you keep calm and pick a topic you are knowledgeable and comfortable with, this can prove to be a very successful station for any candidate.

> **TOP TIP** The medical advancement you choose does not have to be particularly original or groundbreaking, but should be a topic you are comfortable with and can discuss at length.

Even if the interviewer disagrees with you, do not be fazed, but instead appreciate their reasons for disagreement and reply with a balanced answer. Moreover, do not be put off if the examiner is challenging you on many points you raise, as they may simply be pushing you further to see your potential.

Appreciate how this question is worded. It is not asking you to simply list numerous medical advances from the past 200 years, but instead to pick one topic to discuss. Describing a list of medical advances will not gain any credit at this station; they will be looking for you to show other qualities, ranging from scientific knowledge to debating ability.

There are many examples that you could use when tackling this question, some of which include:

- Discovery of antibiotics
  - Since Fleming's discovery in 1928, mass production of antibiotics has saved countless lives from previously untreatable bacterial infections.
- Risks of smoking
  - Led by Richard Doll, the negative health effects of smoking became apparent in the 1950s
  - Since then, mounting evidence has shown the influence smoking has on a variety of diseases, including lung cancer
  - Increasing awareness of this influence has led to an immeasurable number of lives being saved worldwide through smoking cessation.
- Developments in medical imaging
  - The use of radiography in a medical context developed significantly in the 20th century
  - In modern medicine, most hospitalised patients will receive some form of imaging during their stay, aiding the clinical diagnosis significantly.

There are many potential avenues for this question and ensuring you pick a topic you are comfortable with and can discuss well will ensure you achieve highly.

5.8 (T) What is the difference between empathy and sympathy? Do you think it is important for doctors to possess either, and if so why?

The first part of this question requires some knowledge and an ability to articulate what can appear to be a subtle difference:

Empathy: the capacity to understand or imagine the feelings of another from their point of view, often referred to as 'the ability to place oneself in another's shoes'.

Sympathy: also an ability to share the view of another but conveys a sense of pity or sorrow for their misfortune.

The second part of this question is far more subjective. It is important you are able to express and defend your own views. Remember that the interview is trying to test your communication skills and not elicit a 'correct' answer.

I would argue that empathy is an essential skill of a doctor. As a medical student and doctor it is inevitable that you will meet patients who have a very different life to your own, with a different background and different priorities. The ability to appreciate this idea will enable you to more effectively address the needs and concerns of your patients. For this reason empathy is consistently one of the most desired qualities of a doctor. Being able to understand how the patient feels from his or her own perspective and then express that back to them will help you develop the doctor–patient relationship that underpins the delivery of effective medicine. Empathy is also important when thinking about the patient in a 'holistic' manner.

It may be argued that the feeling of sympathy conveys a deep caring for patients, which is another essential attribute of doctors. However, sympathy must not be confused with caring. All doctors should care for all of their patients but they shouldn't necessarily feel sorry for all of them. In fact many patients don't like people to feel sorry for them as they feel it may imply weakness, helplessness or inferiority. At the other extreme some patients may have their recovery hindered if through excessive sympathy they become established in a 'sick role', whereby being ill carries a material benefit. For these reasons I would say sympathy is not strictly necessary although it is likely doctors will often feel sympathetic towards some of the patients they care for.

One may argue that some patients don't necessarily deserve sympathy, given that their illness may be self-inflicted, perhaps through over-eating, smoking or substance abuse. However, one must be very careful not to be judgmental or appear naïve. These patients may have had a traumatic background and have fallen into bad habits against their will or knowledge.

Once you have made your points and created arguments to defend them, summarise with a concluding sentence:

"In summary I would argue that empathy is a vital attribute of a doctor whereas sympathy is more subjective and not strictly necessary or even helpful."

5.9 (MMI) You are asked to propose a research idea to a potential funder. He has £3 million he would like to donate. Please discuss your idea with him and why it should be funded. You can choose any research idea you like. You have 7 minutes.

This question should really make you draw on your personal experience of medicine and any specific interests within it. Some candidates may know exactly how to answer this question, as they might always have had a very clear idea of the specialty they want to pursue, for example:

"I have always been interested in both neuroscience and children's medicine, so ideally I would like to pursue a career as a paediatric neurologist. Therefore, I would want to carry out some further research on paediatric cancers of the brain, specifically neuroblastomas. This is because…"

However, if you don't yet have a specific career in mind, think about your past involvement in medicine. You might have read about a condition or perhaps encountered something interesting while on work experience that you would like to know more about, whether that was with a single patient or a group of patients. Explain what caught your interest and why you would consider spending such a large amount of money in this field.

A good example would be:

"While on my work experience placement at my local GP surgery, I came across a couple of patients who had lupus. Their symptoms really interested me, as they appeared to be quite debilitating at times, and not many patients seemed to present with the same condition. After trying to look further into it in my own time, I realised that lupus is a poorly understood condition in the medical field and so I would like to base my research project around this…"

Remember, although the interviewers don't expect you to have a detailed research plan accounting for every penny, it's probably a good idea to explain roughly what you would spend the money on, so that it's clear that you would be sensible with the funding. It also tells the interviewers that you have some idea of what kind of work goes into a research project, as research is a vital part of medicine and advancements in the field.

Some ideas of how the funding might be used in practice:
- Use of new technology or machinery
- Compensation for participants
- Wages for researchers
- Payment for clinical trials materials e.g. animals, medications

5.10 (MMI) Read the 'abstract' from the following article. What do you think about it? Are there any flaws in the research? You have 10 minutes to read the abstract and 7 minutes to discuss it.

Changes in energy content of lunchtime purchases from fast food restaurants after introduction of calorie labelling: cross sectional customer surveys. Link to article abstract: www.bmj.com/content/343/bmj.d4464

You are not expected to be a research expert. You should use good reasoning to delineate pros and cons of the paper. In answering this scenario, use the following steps:

Comment on the topic

The paper by Dumanovsky *et al.* (*et al.* means 'and others'), published in 2011 in the *British Medical Journal* (*BMJ*) addresses the effect of calorie labelling in restaurants on the buying patterns of customers.

Strengths of the study

The researchers interviewed a large number of people and used multiple restaurants, meaning more viewpoints would have been taken into account. This makes the study relevant to more people. The follow-up period (one year) is lengthy, further adding to the validity of the results.

Weaknesses of the study

This study has a weak research design; there is no 'control' arm and thus one cannot compare the natural trend in calories purchased. It would be better to simultaneously compare the effects on a city where the calorie labelling law is in place to another similar city where the law has not come into force. Factors such as the prevalence of calorie-labelled food before the law was passed, were not taken into account when the results were analysed.

In conclusion

Given the importance of this study in the context of controlling obesity, further studies should be performed before firm conclusions are drawn.

How to analyse a study:

- Is the study qualitative (uses descriptions) or quantitative (uses numbers)?
- Does the question add to the current knowledge base? Is there a flaw in the question?
- Is there an intervention arm and a control arm?
- Are the people in the study typical of the entire population?
- Could the study be biased in the way it has been designed?
- What factors could inaccurately contribute to the results? Does the conclusion acknowledge them?

TOP TIP 'Double-blinded randomised controlled trials' (where patients are divided into two groups, one to which you give the intervention and the other a comparison treatment) are regarded as having a reliable design. Neither the doctor nor patients know which group is which, hence, 'double-blinded'.

Chapter 6 | Questions about medical careers

6.1   *(MMI) You are asked to explain to your fellow applicant some of the pressures of being a medical student, and how you would deal with them. An actor will play the applicant. You have 7 minutes.*

Understanding the reality of being a medical student is crucial for an applicant. The days of full cadaveric dissection, didactic lectures and pre-clinical/clinical split in medicine have largely disappeared from many universities. Integrated curriculums, seeing patients from the first day and problem-based learning are now common and pose different challenges. Familiarise yourself with the medical school's curriculum and tailor your answer accordingly.

This question also provides an excellent opportunity to showcase your experiences with challenges and coping strategies. Divide your answer into two parts, supporting each part with examples.

TOP TIP   Don't forget the question is also testing your communication skills so introduce yourself, check who you are talking to and establish what they know about the pressures of the role already.

Outline the general pressures of being a medical student:
"Medicine has a long training programme with a heavy workload, putting one at risk of burnout. During my A level exam period, I had to balance my prefect duties, as well as sporting and volunteering commitments. During this period I occasionally felt stressed. However, in this period I found taking ten minutes to listen to my favourite music would calm me down. I found talking to my close friends very therapeutic, as they understood how I felt. These techniques have become effective stress-relievers for me and I am well equipped to tackle the academic and extra-curricular commitments of medical school.

The societal pressure to behave in a certain way is unique to medical students. There are certain activities that are considered normal for most other students but which would be unacceptable for a medical student. The General Medical Council (GMC) does offer guidance for medical students and having read the guidance, I feel I will be able to adapt well."

Detail some challenges you expect in the curriculum for the medical school you are being interviewed for:
"At this medical school, students are exposed to patients from week one. This is a completely new experience. My volunteering involves meeting new people every day so I believe I have the ability to communicate well with patients. With my past experiences of working in school projects, I have already begun to develop the skills needed to work effectively in a team. I hope these skills will also help me adapt to the Problem Based Learning sessions."

6.2   (T) What are the disadvantages of a career in medicine?

To ensure that you are making the right career choice, it is the interview panel's role to check whether you are aware of the challenges that doctors can encounter at some point in their careers.

It's a good idea to start off with an opening statement such as:
"I consider medicine to be a highly rewarding, challenging and privileged career. However, I also understand that few, if any, privileges come without disadvantages."

You should now support your statement with examples that help demonstrate your insight into some of the disadvantages of a career in medicine.

"I am aware that a career in medicine will put a considerable demand on my time, which will compete with family and other commitments. It may also involve periods away from family and friends. The combined effect of this, amongst other things, can put a great deal of strain on personal relationships."

Some disadvantages of a career in medicine:
- Competing with family and other commitments
- Strain on personal relationships
- Unsociable hours
- Dealing with uncertainty and risks
- Abusive patients
- Bureaucracy (e.g. discharge paperwork, targets, revalidation, etc.)
- Politicisation of healthcare (e.g. Health and Social Care Act 2012, Government recommendations on pay and working hours, etc.)
- Potential burnout due to stress from a combination of above factors.

It is also a good idea to mention, where possible, how this insight was gained, as it demonstrates evidence of your efforts to research your career choice. For example, perhaps you have asked doctors to share their professional experiences, attended talks on medical careers, used relevant websites, etc.

Finish strongly with a closing statement that puts these back into perspective, e.g.:
"Notwithstanding these points, I am convinced that no career with as great an opportunity to make a real difference to people's lives as medicine comes without sacrifices or stress. I am confident that keeping an honest and realistic view of medicine as a career is the first step towards coping and appropriately dealing with these more negative aspects of the job. I therefore remain very enthusiastic about the prospects of a career in medicine."

Not only will this demonstrate that you possess a well-balanced view of a career in medicine, but it also addresses the potential question: *"Then why pursue a career in medicine?"*

6.3   (T) What have you experienced or read to prepare you for a career in medicine?

There are several things you could have done to prepare yourself for a career in medicine that are worth discussing:
- Speaking to doctors
- Speaking to medical students
- Attending medical school open days
- Work experience in the medical profession or other caring environment
- Attending lectures or workshops on medical careers
- Speaking to a careers advisor
- Doing research into a career in medicine: online, books, journals.

This question is testing whether you have used your initiative to gain insight into a career in medicine. It is also a chance for you to show your enthusiasm and passion for medicine.

A good answer will be one that makes you stand out from all the other candidates. Instead of tediously listing all your work experience, you must deliver your answer in a stimulating manner. You should include how you arranged it (this shows resourcefulness), what you learnt from it and how it prepared you for a career in medicine. Make sure you stick to the questions of how it helped prepare you by using a solid structure. This will ensure that you don't miss anything or waffle. Make it personal by using examples; this will show you have taken the initiative to explore the profession and also adds credibility to your answer. Conclude your answer with a summary of why you are convinced medicine is suited to you.

"I've always been interested in a career in medicine so I decided it would be a good idea to speak to the careers advisor at school. We explored my options and talked about what the career would involve. I then did some research into a career in medicine to learn about what would be required of me. This motivated me to organise some work experience at my local hospital.

I shadowed an obstetrics and gynaecology consultant for a week, which gave me a valuable insight into the profession. It was a great opportunity to see the different roles that a doctor plays, for example communicating with the patient prior to surgery, carrying out the operation and then seeing the patient after the operation. It was inspiring to see many different healthcare professionals working together as a team to ensure the patient received the best care possible. It also demonstrated how much organisation is required to ensure everything goes to plan, which is a skill that I am proud of and look forward to demonstrating in my future career. I really enjoyed speaking to the patient before and after the surgery and hearing about their thoughts and concerns, and I learnt how important it is to fully inform and reassure the patient throughout their hospital journey.

After this week of work experience I was even more eager to get more medical experience and to apply to medical school."

6.4   (T) What do you want to accomplish during your medical career?

This is similar to *Question 3.8*: *"Where do you see yourself in 10 years' time?"* However, it gives you the scope to provide both shorter- and longer-term goals. Think about the different aspects of a medical career and what you would like to achieve in each:

- **Clinical experience:** *"From a clinical point of view, in the short term I would endeavour to become competent in all necessary aspects of medicine. In the long term I would like to become a specialist and at the moment I am interested in immunology. I would like to be able to treat rare diseases and see a real difference in my patients. I am attracted to working in a university hospital in the long term."*

- **Academic:** *"I have always had a passion for teaching, starting from my admiration for my science teacher and then by mentoring Year 7 and Year 8 pupils at my school. I would love to develop my teaching skills and take an active role in teaching within the medical profession. Once I have completed my training I hope to give back to the profession and play a role in training junior doctors. Recently I have taken an interest in reading medical journals and I am inspired by the research carried out. I would love to get involved in research at university and would hope that long term I would be able to work in a team that is making new medical discoveries."*

- **General skills:** *"During my work experience at a variety of hospitals, I learnt about the wide range of skills that are required to be a good doctor; for example, compassion, working within a team and dealing with difficult situations. I hope to build my basic skills in a variety of different areas to ensure I am the best doctor I can be. In the long term I would like to be a consultant with a specialist skill and knowledge area."*

- **Leadership:** *"I enjoy considering how things can be improved and would relish the challenge that a leadership position would bring in the long term. I am inspired by the leadership taken by senior NHS figures such as the President of the Royal College of Physicians and Chair of the BMA and would like to become more involved in these organisations in the medium term."*

- **Personal life:** *"To ensure my medical career is successful and fulfilling I will manage my time so that I can still continue to do my hobbies, such as cycling and reading. I enjoy being academically stimulated but I recognise that it is important to have a balanced work and social life. In the long term I would also like to have a healthy family life with a partner and children."*

Stick to a clear structure so that the interviewer can take in all the points. Then conclude with a summary:
"My teachers and friends have always said that I am very caring and work well within a team. I am keen to use and develop these qualities and to learn new skills throughout my career. I look forward to the many challenges I will face, and, given the chance, I know I will rise to them and strive to achieve beyond them."

6.5   (T) What does a paediatrician spend most of their time doing?

This question is assessing whether you understand the different jobs available to doctors. It would help to know what the common specialties are, such as:

- **Anaesthetics:** Anaesthetists specialise in caring for patients whilst they undergo an operation or when they are critically unwell in the intensive care unit.
- **Cardiology:** Cardiologists treat and prevent heart diseases. They can also perform numerous interventions, e.g. to deploy stents in coronary arteries.
- **Endocrinology:** Endocrinologists treat diseases of the endocrine system, and can prevent patients from developing symptoms related to abnormal hormone levels.
- **Gynaecology:** Gynaecologists treat female patients with problems relating to their reproductive system, e.g. they may remove ovarian tumours.
- **Immunology:** Immunologists treat diseases of the immune system.
- **Neurology:** Neurologists treat diseases related to the brain and the nervous system.
- **Obstetrics:** Obstetricians care for pregnant women and can deliver babies who have difficult births, due to fetal abnormalities or maternal difficulties.
- **Oncology:** Oncologists treat and prevent cancer, e.g. using chemotherapy.
- **Rheumatology:** Rheumatologists treat diseases and abnormalities related to the bones and joints.
- **Paediatrics:** Paediatricians treat babies, children and young people. However, they spend a lot of time counselling, reassuring and explaining information to parents.
- **Psychiatry:** Psychiatrists treat patients who have mental illnesses.
- **Radiology:** Radiologists diagnose and detect physiological abnormalities through the use of imaging technologies. They can also intervene using 'pinhole techniques' guided by X-rays, e.g. to treat patients with diseases in their blood vessels.
- **Surgery:** Surgeons are divided into specialties depending on the area of the body that they focus on. For example, there are cardiothoracic surgeons, neurosurgeons, as well as those who specialise in orthopaedics, ENT (i.e. ear, nose and throat), etc.
- **General practice:** The family doctors who are normally based in the community and are often the first port of call for non-emergencies.

Of course for this specific question you should try to outline the basic aspects of what paediatricians may do:

- Attend clinics to assess new patients (children!), monitor long-term patients and discharge recovered patients
- Go on ward rounds, to monitor patients admitted to their ward
- Prescribe medications
- Paperwork, relating to patient care, referral to other specialists, discharge and follow-up plans
- Attend 'multidisciplinary meetings' to discuss patient care plans with other specialists.

6.6   (T) What is the route to becoming a GP? Describe a typical day for them.

This question is to check how much you know about the various career pathways after a medical degree. Start with the route to becoming a GP:

Becoming a GP takes a total of 5 years after medical school, including:

- Two-year general Foundation training in various specialty rotations
- Three years GP specialist training to achieve a Certificate of Completion of Training or CCT. This length of time may change – ensure you look it up before your interview. During this time trainees spend time in various specialties in the hospital such as 'general medicine', 'emergency medicine' or 'paediatrics'. They will also spend a proportion of time in a GP practice as a trainee GP, performing a role similar to fully qualified GPs.
- You must take the Royal College of GPs exam (MRCGP) before you can start practising as a GP.
- You can then undertake further training to become a GP with a Special Interest (GPwSI) such as mental health or sexual health.

Next, you can go on to describe a typical day, emphasising the variety of the role:
"A typical day for a GP has a lot of variety and patients can present so differently. It may involve a mixture of the following...:"

- Begin the day by liaising with other members of team in a clinic meeting (mention the team you would work alongside, e.g. health visitor, practice nurse, receptionists, community pharmacist, practice manager).
- Next, see patients with various presentations – diagnosing, advising, counselling, prescribing medications, performing minor surgery.
- Patients can present differently and you could be involved in examining a patient, seeing them for a follow-up appointment, explaining how to use an inhaler or a new medication, or counselling someone with a problem.
- Paperwork – making reports, repeat prescriptions, results, arranging blood tests, sending out referral letters.
- Later on you may need to call a few patients who are unable to come in, or do a home visit, or stay for an 'out of hours' clinic.
- If you are a specialised GP, you may run clinics, e.g. skin cancer clinic.

6.7   (T) What do you understand about the role of a nurse?

The main thing in this question is to emphasise:
- Your understanding of their role, with a few examples
- That they are part of the multidisciplinary team working alongside others to provide patient-centred care
- That doctors and nurses often have overlapping roles
- That nurses have differing levels of responsibility and that you are aware they can specialise, e.g. Mental health/Adult/Paediatric, but also with greater responsibility, i.e. nurse practitioners.

You could start with some of their general roles and duties:
- Taking observations and regularly monitoring the patient
- Personal care of the patient
- Administering medication and monitoring their effect – e.g. pain management
- Health promotion – e.g. lifestyle management
- Some nurses are involved in research.

If you have time, you could try to give an example for a few of the roles you have mentioned to help put it into context and really show your understanding.

For example:
"Nurses have a key role in the care of the patient such as regular monitoring of their observations, so that if there are any changes the appropriate course of action can be taken, for instance calling for help or administering pain medication."

You may also want to be prepared for follow-up questions, the answers for which you'll also find in this book, such as:
- Why don't you want to be a nurse instead? (see *Chapter 13*)
- What is a multidisciplinary team? (see *Chapter 14*)

6.8   (T) Describe a day in the life of a junior doctor.

This question is trying to determine what you know about the profession you are seeking to enter. You need to show that you understand the progression through the career and in particular what the job involves.

While the main focus of the question is to see *what* you know it would also be useful to say *how* you know; for example, if you spent a lot of time with a junior doctor on your work experience or if you have discussed with junior doctors whilst researching medicine as career.

Start by showing that you know what a junior doctor is. The term junior doctor is generally used to describe F1 and F2 doctors (foundation doctors). This occurs just after you complete your medical degree and takes two years to complete. (*Technically,* however, all doctors are 'junior doctors' until they complete their specialist training and are eligible to take up a consultant or GP post – potentially ten or more years after graduating!)

You can mention some of the tasks required of a junior doctor:
- Clinical tasks: taking blood, inserting drips, prescribing medication
- Administrative tasks: requesting medical imaging such as X-rays, writing summaries of what care a patient has received in hospital when they are discharged, requesting investigations
- Ward rounds where they review a patient's progress, often with a more senior doctor and nurse
- Working alongside other members of the 'multidisciplinary team' of nurses, senior doctors and other allied health professionals.

You can outline the typical working pattern for a junior doctor:
- It can be long working hours
- Weekend work
- Night shifts.

Whilst you can demonstrate insight by mentioning the effects working such unsociable hours can have on a junior doctor (a difficult social/family life, tiring, etc.), don't forget to mention your motivation: It can be rewarding – this is the first opportunity to make clinical decisions and have the responsibility for patient care. You get to see the direct impact your care can make in the life of a patient!

6.9 (T) Give me an overview of the training pathway to becoming a consultant physician or surgeon.

This question is testing if you have done your background research before embarking on the long career ahead in medicine. You should know this inside out and really show them you have thoroughly thought about what lies ahead.

This is a brief overview of the journey that lies ahead:

*   In the UK medical school is five years but in some universities it is six. This is because students have to undertake a compulsory extra Bachelors degree in addition to their primary medical qualification. When you do this extra degree it is termed 'intercalation'. In medical schools where intercalation is not compulsory, students can still opt to intercalate for a year. Nowadays some universities even let you intercalate in a Masters or doctoral degree.
*   After medical school you do two years as a Foundation Doctor. After your first year as a foundation doctor you will obtain full General Medical Council registration (although this may change in the near future to full registration at the end of medical school).
*   After your foundation years, you will need to enter a training programme and there are a number of options: general practice (GP), hospital medicine (as a doctor working in hospital), psychiatry, obstetrics and gynaecology, a hospital surgeon (a surgeon working in hospital)... You will need to pick one of these options (but not necessarily now!).
*   If you choose to be a hospital doctor or a surgeon you will enter what is called Core Medical or Core Surgical Training. This routinely lasts two years. After these two years you apply into a specialist training programme, e.g. to be a cardiologist or an orthopaedic surgeon. However, there are programmes where you do not have to do Core Medical or Surgical Training first and then reapply. These programmes where you don't need to reapply are termed 'run-through' programmes. Neurosurgery and cardiothoracic surgery are currently 'run-through' programmes. This means you can apply to be a neurosurgeon or a cardiothoracic surgeon straight after Foundation Year 2.
*   Depending on what you pick, the length of training differs dramatically. For example, to become a fully qualified GP takes five years of training after medical school, whereas to become a consultant surgeon takes ten years.
*   After you have successfully completed training in a specialist area, you will be eligible to apply to be a consultant. Remember GPs are not called consultants even though they have completed training. The term 'consultant' is usually only used for hospital doctors and surgeons.

The above is a **very simple outline** of the route to becoming a consultant. Make sure you visit the NHS careers website where there will be a lot of detailed information.

6.10   (T) Where can a medical degree take you?

This is a very broad question! The interviewers want you to demonstrate your knowledge of the breadth of clinical medicine as well as thinking a little 'out of the box'.

Clinical medicine can be split into several large sections, the most obvious split being between primary care (in the community – largely General Practice) and secondary care (in hospitals). This is a good opportunity to show that you are aware of current affairs, e.g. the recent trend towards more 'care in the community' – the proposal to ask patients to visit their pharmacist rather than their GP for everyday minor complaints.

Hospital medicine is divided into many smaller groups, but the majority fall under the headings of 'Medicine' and 'Surgery'. It is not necessary to bore the interviewers with lists of specialties, but you can demonstrate insight by showing that you know surgeons see patients on the wards and in clinic AND operate in operating theatres, or that medics see patients on the wards and in clinic as well as carrying out some procedures such as endoscopy or inserting coronary stents, but do not carry out surgical operations.

Some who qualify from university with a medical degree do not pursue a career entirely (or indeed at all) related to clinical medicine. A medical degree is a great starting point for a career in biomedical research, in medical journalism or in medico-legal affairs. There are several politicians who began their careers working with patients rather than constituents. A medical degree helps to equip you with many transferable skills that stand you in good stead when entering the job market. Many graduate employers look favourably upon the time management and communication skills that must be learnt by all successful medical students. Completing such a long and arduous course also demonstrates one's staying power and steadfastness.

However, whilst medical school comes at a cost to you as the student, the cost to the taxpayer is even more significant. It would therefore be ill-advised to say that your primary goal is to be an MP or a medico-legal specialist. It is much wiser to discuss how you would like a career in clinical medicine and explain all of the other components of such a job, e.g.
- Education
- Research
- Leadership and management, e.g. in a hospital as a medical director, or in a Royal College as a member of their council.

6.11 *(MMI) You are a surgical trainee. You are halfway through an attachment at the colorectal unit of a large teaching hospital. However, you have had very limited opportunity to develop your skills. Discuss this issue with your supervising consultant (played by an actor), explaining the problem and why you feel it is important that you are given the chance to practise your skills. You have 7 minutes to complete this station.*

This scenario is designed to assess your ability to communicate about an issue that is concerning you in a professional manner. Furthermore, it will assess if you recognise the potential risk to patient safety as you progress through your career if you don't receive adequate training. It is important in medicine to speak up if you feel you are not receiving sufficient training opportunities, but you must be able to do so in a very professional manner. (N.B. Surgical training is very much dependent on the opportunity to practise your practical skills, so that you will be able to perform operations independently).

To answer this question:

- Ask your consultant if they are free to talk, and if so, would they mind speaking to you in private.
- Establish a rapport early on by saying that you have enjoyed your placement in the unit so far, but are concerned by certain aspects of it.
- It is important to remain professional and non-confrontational: "*I am annoyed because you aren't letting me do anything in theatre*" is not an appropriate way to address a senior colleague. A more considered way of framing the problem would be to say, "*I am concerned that I am not getting the opportunities I hoped to have in theatre, and I feel this may be impacting on my training*".
- Ask the consultant if there is anything they feel that you can do to improve your learning in theatre, e.g. practising practical skills at home prior to attending theatre or attending extra theatre lists every week. This will show that you are accepting a proportion of the responsibility for your own training, and aren't expecting the consultant to hand you everything on a plate.
- Ask your consultant if they would mind you speaking to them again if you feel the situation doesn't improve.
- Thank the consultant for their time.

6.12 *(MMI) General practice is a 'soft option'. Do you agree with this statement? You have 5 minutes to discuss with the interviewer.*

This is a chance for you to dispel a common stereotypical notion regarding a specialty. You must show understanding of both sides of the argument and provide a conclusion that shows a logical progression from your arguments.

Arguments in favour of the statement:
- There may be less on-call commitment compared to other specialties.
- Care of patients is holistic and not just in an episode of illness.
- The image of the paternalistic family doctor is still present in minds.
- There is an option to work part-time.
- May be seen as a backup option for those not successful in applying to other specialties.
- Seen as 'just a GP' – misconception that general practice is not a specialty in its own right.

Arguments against:
- Must have knowledge of all areas of medicine, not just knowledge in one niche area.
- First port of call for the majority of the general public.
- Varied workload, i.e. seeing patients in practice, on the phone or in their homes.
- Brief and frequent consultations, typically ten minutes each.
- Tremendous responsibility to recognise and refer patients who are seriously ill.
- Physically and emotionally challenging.
- Complexities of a patient's social, home and psychological needs.
- Caring for a patient over the long term, not just for an episode of illness.
- More expertise required than in the past in order to encourage health promotion.

Out-dated stereotypical misperceptions may deter those considering a certain specialty and harm the image of the specialty, resulting in recruitment shortages, as is the case for general practice at present. It may be true that general practice offers a better work–life balance compared to other specialties, but long hours are not the only source of stress in a doctor's working life. In fact as it stands, proposed reforms mean that hours are likely to change in order to achieve a '7-day' NHS.

Contrary to popular misconceptions, general practice offers flexibility and a wealth of opportunities to explore special interests and academia. With the future of healthcare becoming more community-focused as people live longer with more complex management needs, expert generalist care is now needed more than ever and will only be in greater demand in the next decade.

6.13 (T) The Shape of Training Review was set up to look at current UK medical education and training and to provide recommendations for the future healthcare needs of patients. As a future medic, what does it mean to you?

Major changes in workforce planning are required to meet the demands of changing patient demographics and rising co-morbidities. The proposed reforms, in their current state, have been criticised by some major trainee organisations. As a future medic, it is crucial to have an understanding of what these changes mean for current and future medics.

Good points:
- Making training responsive to changing patient demographics and healthcare needs.
- Recommendations of improved mentoring in an apprenticeship-style approach with longer placements and consistent supervision.
- Focus on more general skills in early medical training.
- Improved career advice and more flexible training, allowing doctors to change roles and specialties.
- Moving the point of full registration to the end of medical school (as opposed to the end of FY1, which is currently the case) may allow FY1s the freedom to work throughout the European Union.

Bad points:
- Reduced rotation time on wards, meaning less exposure to ward environment, harming training and competence.
- Changing point of GMC registration to end of medical school, rather than at the end of Foundation Year 1 removes a year of education and experiential training, but graduates are still expected to achieve the same outcomes of safe practice and clinical competence. It also creates additional scope for applicants from EU states to apply to the already oversubscribed Foundation Programme.
- Dangerous and regressive proposed reduction in specialist training time without credible evidence to justify the measures.
- Replacing parts of specialty training programmes with generalist content will adversely impact on the provision of specialist care.
- A well-trained doctor can be a good generalist and a specialist concurrently.
- Implication that more specialists are trained at the expense of generalists is misinformed; in fact a shortage of specialists exists, as exemplified by the length of waiting lists for appointments.
- The number of training posts is to be made dependent on local service needs, thus the field of hospital medicine may become less attractive for ambitious trainees.

6.14 (MMI) "All surgeons are arrogant." Discuss this statement with the interviewer when you enter the interview room. You have 7 minutes.

There is no way to wholly agree with this statement and look good! Essentially you will need to disagree, but you need to talk about why or how this statement might have come about to begin with. Be careful how you phrase your answer – there may very well be a surgeon on your panel of interviewers and they will not take lightly to being criticised in this way!

"I would say that this statement is false and should not be taken as fact. It may, however, be the opinion of a very few individuals..."

Why might someone have stated this? Think about the public's perception of surgeons and how they potentially come across to patients. On the other hand, this statement might also be the opinion of a healthcare professional – have they had negative experiences of working alongside surgeons?

It is important to mention the generalisation in this statement. It may be true that a small number of surgeons do come across in this negative manner. However, this is most likely true in all specialties – within each specific field in medicine, you will find both doctors who come across very positively and also those who do not come across as well.

"The person making this statement may very well have had a bad experience with a surgeon. For example, this might be a nurse who has come across an ill-tempered or unfriendly surgeon whilst trying to manage one of their patients. However, there are probably negative individuals working in all specialties of medicine, rather than just within surgery. On the other hand, there are also many excellent, approachable surgeons, so this statement is probably generalising an entire field based on a minority of experiences."

To offset the negativity portrayed in this statement, you can finish off your answer by talking about ways that surgeons are breaking this stereotype – the fact that there is good team spirit in theatre, excellent communication with patients on ward rounds and the involvement of multidisciplinary teams in patient management. To help you do this, you can draw on your own work experience if you have already had the chance to be present in theatre or work alongside a surgeon.

"My personal experience with surgeons has been the polar opposite to this statement. During my work experience, I got to spend a lot of time in theatre watching procedures, and whilst I was there, the team spirit was really apparent. The surgeons had a good sense of humour as was evident in the team morale and they often praised the other staff members. The surgeons always seemed approachable – staff both inside theatre and out on the wards would come to them without hesitation with questions or comments regarding patients."

6.15 (T) What extra-curricular activities do you undertake and how will these affect your future medical career?

This question is one of the most commonly asked and poorly answered in an interview situation. The reason that medical schools ask this question is to ensure that you can manage your time well and this gives you an opportunity to show off the attributes required of a doctor.

An example of a poor/mediocre answer:
"Outside of school work, I play for the rugby 1ˢᵗ XV team at school. We train twice every day and play every Saturday. We had a challenging game in the final of the county league but eventually won the game 14–12. We played really well and deserved to win the trophy, especially given how hard we trained all season."

Despite describing a great achievement, the above answer fails to show that the candidate is a strong one. It does not highlight any skills that the candidate may have developed; it is not specific about the candidate's role, it makes no reference to a medical career and may even be interpreted as arrogant given the use of the word 'deserved'.

When approaching this question, choose examples that convey your specific contributions and **do not forget to relate your answer back to a career in medicine**. The following example is tailored to show off the skill of *time management*, vital to any medical student. This uses the '**BARL**' technique: **B**ackground, **A**ction, **R**esult and **L**ink to medicine, to illustrate an example:

Background: this sets the context for your extra-curricular activity and what was required of you. *"Outside of school work, I was a member (or even mention a position e.g. fly-half) of the rugby 1st XV team that won the county league trophy. In order to play at my optimal level in the final, I attended training on a daily basis; this forced me to balance my time between mandatory homework and training."*

Action: describes specifically what you did. *"I created a study timetable and discovered that I had three extra hours a week that I could commit to kicking practice after rugby training, without affecting my school work."*

Result: this is the outcome of your activity. *"Owing to my extra practice, my rate of conversion went from 75% to 85% and my kicking won the final game."*

Link: relate your example to medicine. *"The development of a study timetable is a skill that I will use as a medical student and doctor to ensure that I effectively maintain a good work–life balance."*

6.16   *(MMI) A hospital is looking for a new cardiology consultant.*
Using the template provided, fill in the CV of the ideal candidate.
Please explain to the examiner your choices in each section.
You have 7 minutes.

This question is testing your knowledge of the career pathway of a senior doctor. You should know the length and type of training for a medical consultant, surgical consultant and a GP, as described in previous scenarios. This will form the basis of the general requirements for a medical consultant but you should also inform yourself about the specifics of each.

Firstly, you need to know how many years are spent at medical school. This varies between courses for school leavers and those for graduates. The practice of 'intercalation' (taking a year within medical school to study an accelerated undergraduate degree) makes for a stronger CV, as do further studies in the specialty. This could take the form of a Masters, or an MD or PhD (higher degrees in clinical and academic research, respectively).

In the current system, medical training becomes more specialised after the two years spent in the foundation programme. A number of years may be spent in 'core medical' training. Then ensure your imaginary consultant has completed the requisite number of years as a 'specialty trainee' in their field.

In order to practise as a consultant, a doctor must have completed their specialist training and gained their certificate of completion of training (CTT). In addition, they must have passed the exams to become a member (or fellow) of a Royal College. For cardiology, this would be the RCP (Royal College of Physicians). There are equivalent colleges for most other specialties, e.g. Surgery, Paediatrics, Radiology, Psychiatry.

The successful candidate must have a wealth of clinical experience across the specialty, and the skills and knowledge to lead a team of juniors. Playing a leading role in the education of others is an essential requirement. This could be in teaching medical students, junior doctors, or members of other professions. It can take many forms, e.g. leading courses or lecturing for the university.

They may also have performed some research, gained some scientific publications or presentations and carried out some leadership roles.

In the closing personal statement, try to convey a passion for the specialty and give the main reasons the candidate is suited to the job.

Remember, what you choose to enter into the CV of the imaginary successful candidate also gives an insight into the personal qualities you think a doctor needs in order to be successful in their career. Ideally, you should be in possession of these attributes too!

6.17   ***(MMI) You are to talk to a group of GCSE students (played by two actors) about different roles within the NHS. Please use the time to briefly describe the role of the doctor, nurse, physiotherapist, radiologist, occupational therapist, medical physicist and healthcare assistant. You have 10 minutes.***

It is your responsibility to inform yourself about the work of your colleagues in clinical practice. Good team working leads to better outcomes for patients, and you must show respect for the work of the other disciplines.

Remember that you will be talking to younger people, so modify your language accordingly, and use appropriate examples in your explanation.

"There are many different types of job in the NHS. I've been asked to talk to you today about some of the clinical roles. Please let me know if you have any questions as we go through."

As this is an interview for medical school, ensure your understanding of what a doctor does is solid:

"Doctors care for patients by investigating, diagnosing and treating disease. Nurses are involved in the day-to-day holistic care of patients, and will play a role in administering treatments and promoting health in both hospital and community settings."

Show that you have a deeper knowledge of each role than what is commonly known by the general public, reflecting your background research.

"Physiotherapists do not just deal with problems with muscles and bones; they often head up efforts to rehabilitate patients after a period of illness."

Show that you value the work of other clinical professionals by explaining how the role contributes to the health and wellbeing of patients.

"A radiographer is responsible for producing the set of images that will aid in the diagnosis of illness and injury. An occupational therapist may work in primary care, in the hospital or in the community. Their job is to help patients live as independently as possible, using a programme of activities to restore self-sufficiency."

"A medical physicist works to develop and maintain technology used in the care of patients. They may conduct research into new techniques for the diagnosis and treatment of disease. A healthcare assistant aids nurses in the care of patients, and will often get to know patients better than any other professional involved in their care."

Show awareness of the importance of the 'multidisciplinary team' (MDT): *"Each of these roles contributes to multidisciplinary team (MDT) meetings, when a group of specialists work together to ensure all the needs of a patient are met during the investigation, diagnosis and management of disease."*

6.18 (T) Can you tell me about some of the challenges you might face as a doctor?

Doctors can face many challenges. Describing some of these will make your decision to study medicine sound considered. However, it is important not to just list lots of negatives, but to flavour the negatives with your determination to still **study medicine and to see the positive aspects of the career**.

You could begin with a broad statement to make it clear that you have thought about both the pros and cons of the career:
"Life as a doctor is a privilege associated with a rewarding career but there can also be difficulties. From talking to doctors and from what I have seen on my work experience there are a number of potential challenges, for example...:"

- Breaking bad news to patients about a serious diagnosis or poor prognosis can be psychologically draining. But at the same time it is a privilege to care for people in their greatest hour of need.
- Dealing with violent, angry, depressed or demanding patients can be tiring but this is often tempered by the experience of seeing them get better and their mood changing.
- It can be physically demanding work, for example walking for most of the day on a ward or holding a leg up in the operating theatre whilst an operation is carried out. This should be balanced against those who have very sedentary jobs – as a hospital doctor you'll rarely be sitting at a desk all day and this can be a positive.
- It can be smelly: there are lots of bodily fluids on wards! (I can't think of a positive spin to this, other than you still get to do some amazing things despite the smell!)
- Some medical students find the sight of blood extremely disturbing while in the operating theatre. Initially these situations might be difficult, but you often become accustomed to it.

Finish by sounding balanced and considered, but enthusiastic about a career in medicine:
"Though these challenges can be stressful, most doctors learn to manage them over a period of time and I feel strongly that the positives far outweigh the challenges."

Chapter 7 | Communication skills scenarios

7.1 *(MMI) You are a first-year medical student. You are at a small group tutorial with a consultant who is teaching on kidney failure. He asks you what the blood supply to the kidney is. When you explain that you don't know he tells you that you are going to fail the course, he loses his temper and starts shouting at you, telling you that you are stupid. Afterwards, you request a meeting to discuss with him that you weren't happy with how he behaved. Please explain this to the consultant.*

In this station you will be asked to communicate with an actor, who will be playing your consultant. You have 7 minutes to complete this station.

This is a challenging scenario and the interview panel will be assessing how you cope under pressure, how you communicate with someone who is potentially quite angry and how you can communicate something quite challenging to someone who is much more senior than you. A model way to answer this would be:

- **Introduce yourself**: *"Hello, Dr Smith. My name is Akhil Malhotra – I am one of the students who was in a small group tutorial with you."*
- **Build rapport**: *"Thank you for taking the time to teach us – we are very grateful."*
- **Fire a warning shot**: *"However, I wanted to come to talk to you about some of the things that were said during the tutorial."*
- **Stay professional** but state why you were unhappy: *"You mentioned that you thought I was going to fail the course unless I was able to answer the question on kidney failure and kidney anatomy. I was a little concerned about this, as I am quite diligent, and it upset me that it was said with such force in front of my peers."*
- **Maintain rapport and be teachable**: *"I was wondering whether there is anything I could do to improve as I am quite keen to be the best I can be."*
- **Conclude professionally**: *"Thank you for your time and I look forward to our future tutorials."* This is an excellent way to demonstrate that you are teachable, have good communication skills and are able to maintain rapport with someone more senior whilst being able to stand up for what is right.

You will have to maintain a conversation with the consultant as the scenario unfolds but if you follow these steps you will be seen as someone the interview panel would like to work with as a medical student.

7.2 ***(MMI) You have been asked to look after your neighbour's dog. Whilst taking it for a walk you had it off the lead and a car knocked it down. Despite taking it to the vet it has passed away. Please explain this to your neighbour.***
You will be asked to communicate with an actor in this station. You have 7 minutes to complete the station.

The station is testing your ability to break bad news. It also tests your ethics by requiring you to be honest about not having the dog on the lead.

There is a recognised way to break bad news using communication skills and there are a number of different steps that you should follow:

- **Introduce yourself**: This may be unnecessary in this scenario because you have already met the person. Perhaps open with a greeting such as *"Hello, I hope you had a good day trip"* or something similar.
- It is often best to **cut to the chase** when breaking bad news, as opposed to leaving the person hanging on. As such, explaining soon in the conversation is advised.
- **Fire a warning shot** to let the person know that there is some bad news coming. This could take the form of *"I am afraid that I have some bad news..."*
- It is best to explain in **small chunks** what has happened: *"I'm afraid that Rover has died."* Again there is debate about what word to use here (whether we should use the word 'died' or something less harsh such as 'passed away') However, by using the word 'died' you are leaving no doubt in the person's mind about what has happened. This can be important in the initial phase.
- It is best to **leave a short pause** for the person to take the news in at this stage. This can feel awkward for you but can be important for the person to take stock.
- It is best to continue to give the information in small chunks, checking as you go that the person understands what is being said. This could include explaining what happened whilst out walking the dog. It is important in this scenario to also explain that you didn't have the dog on the lead.
- You should **apologise** for not having the dog on the lead as soon as possible and say that you're sorry.
- **Explain** that everything that could have been done was done, including taking the dog to the vet.
- **Explain that you are happy to come back** and see her again or to stay with her this afternoon to make sure she's not on her own.

7.3 **(MMI) *You work in a computer repair shop. The next customer has been waiting in the queue for 30 minutes. She seems very unhappy. She started talking to you with a raised voice and says that this is a terrible company. She explains that she had left her daughter's tablet to be repaired last week. When she got home she found a large crack in the screen, which has left it non-functional. This has resulted in her daughter not being able to complete her coursework for her GCSEs. You have a large queue of customers waiting and have been asked by your boss to speak to this lady, who will be played by an actor in this station. You have 7 minutes to complete the station.***

This scenario tests your ability to communicate effectively with someone who is unhappy. This can occur in medicine. The interviewers will be expecting that you are able to communicate effectively with someone who is upset in a potentially evolving situation.

To deal with this scenario you should follow these steps:

*   **Introduce yourself:** *"Hello, my name is Samantha. I am the assistant at the store today. How can I help?"*
*   **Allow the person time** to explain what has happened and listen. Acknowledge what the person says by nodding your head and perhaps making a sound such as *"Mmm"* to show that you are being empathetic.
*   If the person is shouting, **invite them to a quieter part of the store** to avoid upsetting other customers.
*   After **listening**, use a phrase such as *"I'm **sorry** that you are upset, and I'm sorry that the service has not been up to the standards that you expect."* This doesn't admit that you've done something wrong but does acknowledge the fact that the person is upset.
*   **Explain how you will solve the problem.** This might mean taking the tablet to have a look at what has happened and offering a repair.
*   **Do not rise to the person's anger.** You can use a technique called 'mirroring' to help reduce the person's aggressive behaviour. This involves mirroring their behaviour initially, e.g. standing in a similar position to them, and then gradually becoming more relaxed. The theory is that this reduces the person's aggressive behaviour.

This is a common scenario in healthcare and whilst we don't deal with tablets or computers we deal with families, patients and their loved ones. Occasionally the system does perform poorly and it's important to provide the person with an apology, an explanation if possible, an action plan about what you are going to do to rectify the problem and a source for making a further complaint if necessary. Each hospital has a patient advice and liaison service to provide that support.

7.4   *(MMI) You are a medical student. Two patients are in the waiting room in the accident and emergency department. One is a 75-year-old patient who has had chest pain and was found collapsed at home. The second is a 25-year-old man who has a painful finger after slamming it in a door by accident. The man with a painful finger is angry because he has been kept waiting and has just been told that the other patient will be seen first. All of the other staff in the accident and emergency department have been called away to another patient who is exceptionally unwell. You are asked by the receptionist to discuss with the angry patient and explain to him why the other man will be seen first. You will be asked to communicate with an actor in this scenario. You have 7 minutes to complete this scenario.*

This is a complex scenario that requires not only exceptional communication skills but also the ability to decide upon which patient is more ill.

Deciding upon why the other patient is to be seen first is probably the first decision that you have to make. To do this you have to recognise the fact that the man with chest pain is potentially very ill, possibly unstable and requires more urgent treatment. If the man who has slammed his finger in a door doesn't have any other problems going on he should be seen second.

Now to communicate the decision:
- **Introduce yourself**: *"Hello, my name is Sophie and I am a medical student."*
- If the patient is particularly loud **invite him away from the main waiting room** to avoid making a scene. Talking with him individually would also maintain patient confidentiality.
- **Establish patient identity** and why they have come to hospital – make sure that they haven't had a change in their condition.
- **Explain to the patient that there may be a short wait** for treatment. Explain why this is the case: that there are other sick patients and we have to treat people by priority of medical need. **Apologise** for the wait.
- **Reassure** him that he will be seen.
- Explain that if he remains unhappy you can **let the doctor/nurse know when they become available**.
- **Be polite and courteous.** Remember that this is a test of your communication skills – listen, remain calm and allow the person to speak, and don't become angry or raise your voice.

7.5 *(MMI) You are working at a general practice clinic in your summer holidays. Your job is to answer the telephone. The next phone call you receive is from a private company who sell gym memberships. They request that you provide the names, telephone numbers and addresses of all patients within the practice who are overweight or have had obesity treatment. Please discuss this with them as you see fit.*

You will be asked to communicate with an actor on the telephone in this station. You have 7 minutes to complete the station. To start the station: pick up the telephone and dial 2059.

This is a question that tests your ethics, your understanding of confidentiality and your communication skills.

- Begin by **introducing yourself**: *"Hello, my name is Neel and I am the practice receptionist."*
- **Ask how you can help them** and find out exactly who they are. This might involve taking the company name, the name of the person you are speaking to and how you can get back in touch with them (telephone number and address).
- After they make their request, **explain to them** that you would be unable to provide that information.
- Explain why you are unable to provide the information, including the importance of **confidentiality** of your patients.
- They may attempt to pressure you into giving information and it is important that you **do not give in to this pressure**.
- It would be worth **raising this request with one of your senior colleagues** (this may be one of the doctors in the practice). Whilst if you were in a real-life setting you may not say this on the telephone, it may be worth saying it in the scenario because otherwise you may not demonstrate that you know that this is important. A comment which would help you get this point across might be: *"Just to let you know I am going to let the GP partners in the practice know about this request and if they have any further questions they can then contact you."*
- Ask if there is anything else you can help with.
- Close the conversation with *"Thank you, goodbye."*

7.6 **(MMI) You work for a Member of Parliament. Prior to a vote on the introduction of a new smoking ban in cars carrying children you have a conversation with one of the constituents. She would like to know the pros and cons of banning smoking in cars containing children. She has also been told there will be a referendum on the topic and would like to know what way she should vote if this happens.**
You will have 2 minutes to prepare your thoughts and 5 minutes to address the constituent and answer her questions. You will be asked to communicate with an actor in the station.

This question is testing your ability to think logically about a topic, be able to give information and communicate effectively with a member of the public.

The conversation should follow a logical sequence to allow you to develop your thoughts as well as address the concerns of your constituent:

- **Introduce yourself.** Find out who they are. Ask something like *"How can I help?"*
- When addressing their query about smoking in cars you should **establish what they understand already**, *"What do you already know about the proposed change to the law?"* This allows you to base your answers on meeting their needs.
- In answer to the person's query explain that there are pros and cons (see below).
- Provide **small chunks** of information at a time and check that the person understands each point as you give it.
- Whilst there hasn't been and probably won't be a referendum on this topic you should play along with the scenario. It is testing your ability to appreciate that the voter has the right to 'autonomy' – to make their own decision. You can only provide pros and cons. This is very similar to making decisions in healthcare: patients should be allowed to make an informed decision and should not be pressured.
- **Summarise** your conversation. Conclude by asking if you can help with anything else.

Pros of a ban on smoking in a car carrying a child:
- Protects young people from the negative effects of passive smoking.
- Reduces children's observation of smoking and makes the behaviour less normal.
- Helps adults to focus on driving and reduces the number of road traffic accidents.
- May reduce the number of cigarettes smoked by adults and improve their health.

Cons of a ban on smoking in a car carrying a child:
- The ban may violate free will.
- It may result in agitated drivers who have not had a cigarette in a number of hours.
- It may be difficult to police and therefore undermine the rule of law.
- There aren't many scientific studies to say that the ban will make any difference to child health or to the number of people who will be saved from lung cancer.

7.7 *(MMI) You are a medical student on a ward and are asked to discuss with a patient about her hospital admission – find out about why she came to hospital, how she has been treated and any other relevant information.*
Please discuss with her. You will be asked to communicate with an actor in the station. You have a total of 5 minutes to complete the station.

You have already been asked to PROVIDE information in other questions in this section. This question is testing your ability to GATHER sensible information. It is almost beyond a medical school interview scenario, and as such would be one of the more challenging questions you could receive. You will not be expected to perform at the level of a medical student – it is more to check that you can think on your feet and ask sensible questions.

- Introduce yourself and ask if it's OK to talk about why they are in hospital, i.e. get 'consent' from the patient.
- Find out the patient's name and date of birth.
- The next part of the conversation has a structure when you are a doctor – you will not be expected to know what it is, but it's actually fairly sensible and by telling you now, it will hopefully help you ask some logical questions if you are faced with this sort of scenario:
    - **'History of presenting complaint'**: i.e. why the person came to hospital: what were their symptoms, how were they feeling, what was going on – was it pain, vomiting, diarrhoea, weakness, breathlessness? Find out a time frame – did it happen suddenly or gradually, has it been happening on a regular basis or is this the first time it's happened? Ask if they have any other symptoms they want to tell you about. You won't be expected to know what symptoms to ask about, so keeping the questions quite wide and open is advised.
    - **'Past medical history'**: i.e. does the person have any other health problems?
    - **'Drug history'**: Does the person take any medication? Do they have any drug allergies?
    - **'Family history'**: Is there anything that runs in their family?
    - **'Social history'**: Find out more about the person – what do they do for a living? Do they smoke? Do they drink alcohol? Who do they live with?
    - Find out about **what their time in hospital has involved**: have they had any tests done? What treatment have they had? How long have they been in hospital? What is the plan going forward?
- Ask if there is anything else they want to tell you.
- Summarise what you have found out back to the patient.
- Thank them and close the conversation.

7.8 ***(MMI) You are a medical student. You are asked to answer a surgeon's phone whilst they are busy. Listen to the information given to you and tell the surgeon about it when they are free. You are provided with a piece of paper and a pen to make notes if you require. You will be asked to communicate with an actor in the station. You have 3 minutes to read and make notes on the transcript and 4 minutes to relay the information to the actor. Transcript (words in brackets are explanations of terms):***

"Hello, it's Tom the registrar in A&E. We have an 85-year-old man who has come in today with a 4-hour history of severe epigastric [upper central abdomen] pain. He has been vomiting and has been feverish. He has a past history of arthritis for which he takes oral steroids and non-steroidal anti-inflammatories. He doesn't have any allergies. He also has hypothyroidism and inflammatory bowel disease. His social history includes alcohol excess and smoking 20 per day. He has a family history of bowel cancer and gastric cancer. On examination he is tender in the epigastric area and his abdomen is rigid. His lungs are clear and have good air entry and his heart sounds are normal. His heart rate is high at 110 beats per minute and his blood pressure is low at 90/60. He is pyrexial [has a temperature]. We've got an erect chest X-ray, which doesn't show any free air under his diaphragm but his inflammatory markers are elevated in his bloods. I think he might have a perforated stomach ulcer and so have started antibiotics and fluids. He may need an operation."

This question is testing your ability to accurately relay important information. You have been offered a pen and paper so make use of it!

- **Introduce** yourself to the surgeon.
- There is a way to convey a message to people that allows you to explain exactly what has happened in a clear and logical way: it's called **SBAR – Situation, Background, Assessment, Recommendation.**
  - **Situation**: Explain that you have had a phone call from A&E, who it was from and explain that they wanted to refer a patient who might need an operation.
  - **Background**: Explain the patient's name and age. Explain that they have come in with upper abdominal pain and their tummy is rigid and tender in the upper abdomen.
  - **Assessment**: They have a blood pressure of 90/60, a heart rate of 110 and they have a temperature. They have done a chest X-ray that didn't show "free air under the diaphragm" and his bloods show raised inflammatory markers. They think he has a perforated stomach ulcer.
  - **Recommendation**: They wanted to talk to you about whether they need an emergency operation.

The surgeon may also ask you about some other bits of information, so ensure that you listen to the phone call carefully. Remember to be honest if asked a question to which you haven't been provided with an answer. It is better to be honest and say *"I don't know"* or *"The doctor in A&E didn't tell me that"* than to risk hurting someone.

7.9 *(MMI) You have been asked to prepare a 2-minute presentation to local primary schoolchildren on the benefits of healthy eating. Please prepare a short talk and deliver this to the two actors. They will then ask you questions about your presentation. You will NOT have a computer or slides available. You have a pen and paper to use as you wish.*

You have 12 minutes to prepare your thoughts, 2 minutes to deliver your presentation and 2 minutes for questions – a total of 14 minutes to complete the station.

In medicine your communication skills are required not only to communicate with patients and relatives but also to colleagues in an individual and group setting. This station is testing your ability to present to a group.

To do this you require two things:

1. The ability to develop a talk on the topic you have been given – this means you might have to think outside the box
2. Presentation skills.

To answer this question:

- **Introduce yourself** briefly.
- **Outline the objectives** of your talk (in such a short talk a single objective or two objectives may be suitable since you don't have much time). Remember who your audience is and pitch it at the right level!
- **Establish what the learners know already.** Perhaps ask a question: *"Do you eat healthily?"* or *"What is the healthiest thing that you ate yesterday?"*.
- **Explain what is meant by healthy eating.**
- **Explain what foods are healthy**, e.g. fruit and veg, fibre, lean meats. Explain that a diet should be balanced to contain a variety of food items.
- **What are benefits of healthy eating?** Less heart disease, fewer strokes, less chance of diabetes, longer life...
- **Briefly summarise** what you have discussed: *"So we have talked about what foods are healthy and what the benefits are."*
- Invite **questions**.

7.10 **(MMI) You are in a problem-based learning group. Your fellow coursemate has come to each of the previous ten sessions, and hasn't participated in the conversation. Further, when people are talking he will be writing down everything other people are saying. You don't feel he is pulling his weight. Your fellow students have nominated you to discuss this with him. Please discuss with the actor as if he is the medical student who is not pulling his weight. You have a total of 7 minutes to complete the station.**

This is a challenging scenario because you have to communicate with a coursemate who perhaps your group feels slightly resentful of. You should remain professional, without compromising your message to the student. A helpful way to answer these scenarios might be:

- **Introduce yourself.** Ensure you have the correct person – this might be slightly false in this situation but demonstrates that you know that this is an important part of communication skills.
- **Explain why you are there to talk to him** today in a general sense: for example thanking him for coming in and explaining that you would like to discuss the PBL group.
- **Begin by finding out how he finds the group.** Perhaps he recognises that he has been struggling?
- **Explain that you have noticed that he is not keeping up with the tasks set by the group.** You can maintain rapport with him by explaining that you are concerned about this and wonder if there is anything going on that could be causing it – "*Is everything OK at home?*" "*Are you finding the course challenging?*"
- Use your **initiative** to help in the situation. Could you assign tasks to each group member? Could you recommend a good course textbook? If it's problems at home can you help? Could you request that all group participants email their notes to the facilitator the night before the meeting?
- If there are personal problems or if the student's performance still doesn't improve it would be worth **highlighting this to your tutor**. Explain your intentions to do this to your coursemate in a sensitive way.
- Remember to **be encouraging**: explain that if you can help him in any way just to let you know.
- **Thank him.**

7.11 *(MMI) You are a student at a university in the south of England. You are on a night out with some friends. On your way home you walk across a bridge high up above the city gorge. You notice someone acting suspiciously on the bridge and you hear them crying. You decide to talk to them. You will be asked to communicate with an actor in the station. Please have the conversation with the actor as if they are the person who is crying on the bridge. You have a total of 7 minutes to complete the station.*

This is a scenario that requires you to be perceptive. It is likely to involve a discussion around low mood. This is important because some of your patients will have symptoms of depression and you will have to develop a way to communicate with them. In this specific scenario you are asked to speak to someone who is potentially thinking about jumping off the bridge. In these circumstances it would be wise to get some professional help – there are emergency and voluntary services staff who are specially trained to help in these situations. You need to be both friendly and sensitive.

- Open the conversation with a gentle comment, *"Hello, I'm Jack. I was walking past and heard you crying. Is everything OK?"*. The person is likely to answer with either: *"Yes – leave me alone"* or be honest about why they are crying. Either way you should offer them some help.
- If you have a friend with you, you might want to ask them to get some help early in the encounter, to allow you to stay with the person. Ringing the emergency services in the first instance would be advisable. If you don't have a friend with you, which is likely to be the case during the interview, you will have to call for help yourself. If so, you may have to call the emergency services in front of the person. Take into account that they might not like the idea of emergency services getting involved.
- Listen. If they start to explain how they are feeling you should provide time for the person to talk to you. Make sure you listen and don't butt in to offer solutions. Simply listening to the person is often quite powerful.
- If there is something practical you can do to build rapport, do it, e.g. *"You look so cold – would you like my coat?"*
- Offer the person an option to come away from the bridge, e.g. *"Would you like to get a hot drink?"*
- Offer some hope. This will depend on the reason for their being on the bridge but encouraging them to think about something positive they have mentioned may help: their child of whom they are proud, a new job, their partner whom they love...
- If you have ever been in the situation the person is currently in, talk about your experience with them.

This is going to be a challenging scenario and would be one of the more difficult ones you could receive. Remember to remain calm, listen and don't give up – stay with the person at least until you get help from the emergency services.

7.12   *(MMI) You are on a ward round as a medical student and smell alcohol on the breath of one of your coursemates. He is about to take blood from a patient. Please communicate with him.*
You will be asked to communicate with an actor in the station.
You have a total of 7 minutes to complete the station.

This raises a number of issues and a good way to approach the person is:

- Introduce yourself.
- Ask him to step outside the ward for a few minutes. Don't confront him in front of a patient unless he refuses to leave the ward.
- Ask him whether he has been drinking. He may deny it. Either way you should explain that you could smell alcohol on his breath.
- Explain that you will have to tell the consultant supervisor what has happened and that he should stay in the staff room until the consultant comes to see him.
- Explain that this is quite serious and the consultant is likely to ask him to go home without seeing any more patients. It is not safe to be treating patients when you have had a drink of alcohol. Even if it is from the night before, it is still quite serious. It demonstrates a lack of judgment and little respect for patient safety.
- Ask if he has a safe way to get home – bus, train or taxi. Make sure that he doesn't drive home!
- There may be a personal reason why he was drunk in hospital. Is there a problem at home? Is he struggling with the course? Make sure you are not judgmental – and instead offer support if there are personal problems. Would he like to come over for a cup of tea at your house to discuss?
- Get some senior support early – don't deal with this situation on your own!

7.13   **(MMI) You are a medical student in clinic. You are asked to discuss with a patient about their upcoming gallbladder operation. The patient is overweight. You are asked to explain to them that they are overweight and they should lose weight before the operation. If you can, please explain why this might be important. You will be asked to communicate with an actor in the station. You have a total of 7 minutes to complete the station.**

This question is testing your ability to be tactful but still able to communicate clearly. It is not easy to tell someone they are overweight and must lose weight, but it is important.
- Start by introducing yourself.
- Find out what they know already – has someone told them that they are having an operation and that you are going to discuss some things regarding that?
- Ask the person if they feel there is anything they think they should do or give up before the operation – it is made easier if the person tells you that they feel they are overweight!
- If they don't volunteer the information you could gently explain that you have spoken to the surgeon who feels that **for their own safety** it is important that they lose some weight before the operation. By explaining it in this manner it makes it sound more acceptable to the patient. They will feel you are not being as judgmental as if you just said, *"You're going to have to lose some weight"*.
- It is likely that they will ask *"How much weight?"*. If you are unsure, it is important to say this and say that you will check with the operating surgeon. This demonstrates that you are honest and know your limits.
- If you know why it is important to lose weight say this. If not, try to work it out – it may require you to think on your feet:

  Losing weight helps:
  - prevent breathing problems after/during the operation
  - with healing
  - prevent clots in legs and lungs (DVTs – like you might get on a long–haul flight)
  - make minimally invasive surgery easier – less depth of fat until you get into the abdomen.

- Summarise the conversation and check the person understands.
- Thank them and shake their hand.

7.14 *(MMI) You will be asked to discuss the ethics of euthanasia with a group. Please consider the pros and cons of euthanasia as well as the ethical issues it raises. You will be assessed on your ability to work as part of the group, how much you contribute to the discussion, whether you articulate your thoughts clearly and how much you take into consideration other group members' points of view. You will be asked to communicate with a group. You have a total of 7 minutes to complete the station.*

You are being assessed on how well you can communicate with a group. This will test if you can strike a balance between speaking too much and not participating. The goal is to not shy away from group discussion, but also not to be overbearing.

Some tips to get on well in a group:
- Ask questions
- Ask people for their opinions
- Don't speak all the time
- Don't remain quiet
- Look at people when they talk
- Don't be overbearing when you share your opinion
- Pick up on what other people say and incorporate it into your answer
- Involve the quieter group members.

Some pros of euthanasia:
- Allows people to die with dignity
- Alleviates suffering
- Removes the cost of caring for people who don't want to remain in a vegetative state – controversial!

Some cons of euthanasia:
- Involves doctors in the role of killing people
- It may be a slippery slope and encourage blurred ethical boundaries
- May negatively impact on the doctor–patient relationship with other patients.

7.15 *(MMI) You are a member of a problem-based learning group. Four members of the group have been asked to debate the pros and cons of offering a 14-year-old an abortion. You are asked to be pro-abortion in this situation along with another group member. Two other group members will be anti-abortion in this situation. Debate the situation in a professional manner, speaking for a maximum of 2 minutes each. You will be asked to communicate with a group.*

This is a test of how you will get on in a PBL group with an assigned task. It requires you to think logically, and potentially to argue a point of view which isn't necessarily your own. This requires you to think outside the box and appreciate other people's thoughts.

Remember to remain professional and to make only factual or well-constructed arguments – don't resort to personal comments!

Some points you might want to consider:

Pro abortion in this scenario:
- The girl might find the process of giving birth psychologically distressing
- The baby may not be happy growing up 'unwanted' or adopted
- The girl may drop out of school to care for the child or there may not be an adult suitable to look after the child in the family
- The girl has a choice of what to do with her own body and that should be protected.

Against giving the girl an abortion:
- She may not be mature enough to make that decision
- She may suffer physical harm due to the abortion
- The baby may be quite healthy and live a normal life even if adopted by someone else
- The abortion may be psychologically scarring as well as physically
- The baby should have a right to be protected.

7.16 **(MMI) It is your son Tom's first birthday party. You have been planning the event for weeks. However, you are the consultant surgeon on call and there has been a stabbing. The patient is in a critical condition and is bleeding profusely. You have received a telephone call asking you to come in to the hospital to remove the knife and stem the bleeding. Please explain to your spouse what you are going to do. You have 7 minutes. An actor will play your spouse.**

Situations like this can be extremely emotive. If you are the consultant on call it is important that you attend the emergency. Whilst neither your spouse nor child may welcome this, it is inappropriate and unprofessional to neglect your duty as the surgeon on call.

This scenario is similar to other scenarios where you have to break bad news. You must explain the gravity of the situation to your spouse and explain why it cannot wait. It may help to apologise to them and to explain how this situation might be avoided in the future.

Begin by showing that you understand how important the birthday party is:
"I realise that today is a very important day for Tom and that we have been planning this for weeks."

Fire a warning shot that you have some bad news:
"Although, unfortunately I have some really bad news."

Then explain, concisely, what has happened and why you must leave:
"I've had a telephone call from the hospital. There's a young man who has been stabbed, and is bleeding profusely. He's in a critical condition. I've been asked to go in to operate on him. It sounds like this is a case of life or death."

Apologise:
"I'm so sorry."

Your spouse may be upset because this is an important day in your lives. They may be frustrated because it has happened before (a very real prospect as a doctor!). They may, however, be understanding and be in full support of what you must do. It is likely if this scenario is used that the spouse will be frustrated or upset because this will be a greater test of your communication skills.

Explain that you *"hope to be back as soon as possible"* and it may be helpful to explain that you will ensure Tom receives another celebration with you soon.

It may also be helpful to say how you will prevent this from happening in the future, e.g.
- asking a colleague to cover your shift in advance of important dates
- ensuring your spouse knows the dates you are on call well in advance.

Chapter 8 | Problem-solving scenarios

8.1 **(MMI) You are a doctor working in the NHS. Swine flu has become a fatal epidemic. The hospital is very busy and under-staffed. You are due to go to work; however, a member of your family is now unwell with swine flu. Please explain to the interviewer what you would do. You have 5 minutes to do so.**

The interviewers will want to know your thought processes and reasoning behind everything you say in response to this question.

Beginning the answer

Take a few seconds to think about how you are going to address this question. Don't feel the need to rush into an answer; a short pause will also make you come across as thoughtful, and this is much better than digging yourself into a hole with a hasty answer.

You should acknowledge that it is a tough question, with a brief comment such as *"This is a very difficult situation"*.

First of all you need to address the dilemma

You have a duty as a doctor to go to work and to look after patients. However, you also feel like you should be with your family member during this difficult time, and you could potentially also now be infected. Whatever you say, it is important to back it up properly and offer a solution.

What would happen if you want to stay at home?

The hospital is short-staffed, not surprisingly given there is an ongoing crisis. Therefore, if you do not go into work, the team will be under tremendous pressure, and the quality of care to patients will be compromised. You have a duty of care to patients as a doctor and an obligation to go into work as a professional.

You should warn work that you have been in contact with someone with swine flu and seek urgent advice on whether it is safe or appropriate for you to go to work. If you want to stay at home to care for your family member you should try to help by finding a colleague who would be willing to cover for you at work. If this is not possible you could try to think of other reasonable solutions. Perhaps your family member may even need to go to hospital, given her illness. Could that mean you go for your shift and ask colleagues if it is OK to visit her once every couple of hours?

It is very likely that the interviewers will not accept a vague answer. This is because they want to see how you react under pressure. So long as you can support whatever final decision you have come to, it is fine to say what you believe is the right thing to do.

8.2 (MMI) The European Working Time Directive has limited the amount of time that junior doctors work, and therefore the amount of time they spend on the wards caring for their patients. Explain to the interviewer, in 5 minutes, how you would maintain continuity of care in light of this fact.

The European Working Time Directive is a piece of EU legislation, used to ensure that no EU citizen has to work more than 48 hours a week on average. Initially, junior doctors were not covered by this legislation, due to concerns regarding training, but were eventually included in 2008.

This question aims to test your knowledge of issues related to training and service delivery in medicine, how they impact on patient care, and the importance of adequate handover (communication between healthcare professionals is vital to ensuring important information about patients is known to those looking after them).

You should begin by demonstrating that you know more about the European Working Time Directive than has been revealed in the question, to show that you have read around the topic and keep up to date with issues relevant to medical practice.

"I am aware that the European Working Time Directive is an EU law, introduced to limit the hours an EU citizen works to an average of 48 hours a week, that was extended to cover junior doctors in 2008. I know that it has caused some problems regarding opportunities for training, particularly in surgical specialties."

Following this introduction, you should now establish that you appreciate the potential difficulties this legislation could cause for continuity of care, and what you would do to tackle them.

"Junior doctors working fewer hours leads to more frequent changes in the staff looking after a patient, making communication between the different members of staff hugely important to patient safety. In order to facilitate effective handover, I would ensure that I spoke to the member of the staff caring for my patients before they finished their shift, taking a note of any particular issues and ensuring I clarified anything I was unsure of before beginning my shift."

8.3 (T) What challenges and opportunities does social media provide for physicians?

This question is testing your ability to debate the use of social media, its appropriateness, and the opportunities it offers. You must present both sides of the argument and keep to a central focus, i.e. patient trust in the profession.

Social media has a dominant presence in our everyday lives. It allows physicians to connect, share, learn and support each other. However, maintaining responsible online conduct and professionalism are key to reaping the immense benefits it offers.

Challenges:
- Overwhelming and continuous stream of information available online
- User-generated content lacks clearly defined quality control
- Reader responsible for deciding the credibility of available information
- May potentially violate patient confidentiality; more serious online due to the potential wide reach and permanency of content posted
- Serious damage to physician's career or their institution's reputation
- Boundaries between personal and professional content online are blurred
- Professional character judged on the basis of online behaviour and presentation.

Opportunities:
- Sharing credible health information and resources
- Facilitating communication with patients to augment health promotion
- Disseminating research and other health information, e.g. using hashtags such as 'FOAMed' and 'MedEdTips' (search for them on Twitter!)
- Combating the powerful voice of media that may be spreading misleading and inaccurate statements about health
- Communicating and networking with peers
- Learning aid for students and physicians for continuing professional development
- Telemedicine (e.g. virtual clinics) can help reduce health disparities in rural areas
- Used by international medical relief organisations to communicate with those working in remote areas and helping coordinate medical and logistical demands.

Responsible use of social media offers a great wealth of opportunities, but as the use of social media in clinical care grows, so must physician awareness about its impact on our ethics and profession. It is for this reason that organisations such as the British Medical Association and General Medical Council have published guidelines regarding use of social media.

8.4 (T) People can buy medicines online, including many products that are prescription-only in the UK. Discuss the associated dangers.

Consider the different ways in which the online purchase of drugs can be dangerous; take a few minutes at the start to formulate your thoughts and divide your answer into a few key points in order to keep it coherent.

Facilities to purchase drugs without prescription were already available before the advent of the internet, in the form of mail order or advertisements in magazines, but the searchable option provided by the internet and the ease of access means that these products are available to purchase with much greater ease. Purchasing pharmaceuticals online can be convenient and possibly cheaper, but there are a multitude of risks that may be associated with this practice:

Quality of pharmaceuticals:

- There is a danger that fake, sub-standard or even harmful medicines may be purchased.
- New drugs that have not yet been properly tested or approved may also be available for purchase online.

Appropriateness of medication:

- Medicines may not be what they purport to be.
- They may be masking symptoms rather than treating the underlying condition.
- There may be incomplete information about adverse effects and contraindications.
- There is a risk of harmful interactions with other medication the patient is already taking.
- Pharmaceuticals purchased from foreign sources may have different names and labels, leading to confusion.
- Access to antibiotics without prescription may further contribute to antibiotic resistance and this could have a serious impact on public health.

Doctor–patient relationship:

- Drugs may be bought without consulting health professionals who take the patient's entire case into account.
- Websites that are not a registered pharmacy cannot offer advice regarding the use of medication for the individual concerned.
- Patients may inadvertently select the wrong form or dosage, as unlike prescriptions, online orders are not rechecked by nurses or pharmacists.
- There are no limits on quantity purchased, thus risking overdoses.
- Consultation with health professionals may be deferred, and this could lead to delayed diagnosis or deterioration in the treatment.

In the UK, legislation exists that prevents the sale of drugs by unregistered agencies, or of unlicensed drugs. Those who breach these rules are criminally liable and may face severe penalties for a repeated offence. The General Pharmaceutical Council imposes strict standards for registered pharmacies wishing to trade on the internet, but these only apply within the UK.

8.5 (T) What problems are associated with patients using the internet for medical information?

The internet is a widely available, convenient and valuable resource. Information regarding health can be empowering for patients, helping them understand their medical condition and improving self-care, thus reducing the burden on the NHS. They can also use the internet to find support through discussion groups and forums, as well as to chronicle their illness journey via social media. However, when not used appropriately, it can be conflicting and overwhelming. Other issues with medical information found online include:

- Information may not be reliable as it does not go through an editorial process and the source may not be cited.
- If information is found on blogs/community posts, it may only be subjective accounts of individual patients, and thus not necessarily medically accurate.
- It may be too complicated or contain too much jargon for a layperson to understand.
- Information may be outdated or irrelevant.
- Misleading information may cause unnecessary anxiety for the patient.
- It may possibly lead to inappropriate self-diagnosis.
- Patients may wish to try a non–conventional, possibly dangerous treatment that they discover via the internet.
- Limited consultation times can be made even more challenging by questions arising from information obtained from the internet.
- If the patient's choice of treatment is at odds with the doctor's expert opinion, it may adversely impact the doctor–patient relationship.

A patient accessing the internet to get information regarding their health problems is inevitable. However, in order to ensure patient safety, a number of methods can be employed during consultations:

- Assisting patients in evaluating the quality of medical information on the internet.
- Recommending reliable and accurate health information websites, such as NHS Choices.
- Informing patients about specific relevant health websites and organisations that provide expert advice and information, such as Stroke Association or British Heart Foundation.

Ultimately, always recommend that the patient consult a healthcare professional regarding their concerns about health issues.

8.6 (T) Describe some of the typical problems you might face on a daily ward round as a junior doctor.

To answer this question, ideally, you will have had some experience of working in a hospital environment, as the problems you could face become really apparent while you're actually in this situation.

Problems can vary depending on the level of doctors involved – for example, an FY1 is likely to have different priorities than a senior consultant. However, largely, it's the same sorts of issues that crop up again and again. These include:

- Time – usually there is not enough of this to get everything done!
- Completing paperwork – a necessary task that is required by law but which may get in the way of patient care...(an interesting debate for another day!)
- Prioritising patients – acute patients are usually seen first, but this could mean patients with chronic co-morbidities being continually left until last, which could potentially extend hospital stay.
- Attendees – with medical students, various levels of doctors and different types of nurses/therapists, there can be as many as seven or eight people standing around the bedside, so think about how this might seem for the patient.

You can really emphasise your personal experiences of being in the hospital environment when answering this question. If you have been lucky enough to experience ward rounds in different wards/parts of the hospital, comparing and contrasting the different places will impress the interviewers, as it shows reflection and awareness of your surroundings. What problems came up in both areas? Did one of the wards have a more specific problem and why was this?

Of course, it is always helpful in an interview to finish by talking about how you would tackle these problems – it shows the interviewer that you have what it takes to be a future medic! For example:

"However, although there may be various issues that arise during a ward round, I feel that in the past I have demonstrated the skills necessary to deal with any potential problems. I have shown that I have good time management skills during my time in sixth form – this will enable me to see all my patients and complete all ward round tasks in the time allotted. As well as this..."

8.7 ***(T) Suppose you have three tasks of equal importance. Firstly, you have a shift at work today, but your child is ill and you need to take them to hospital, and you also have to hand in a report tomorrow to your supervisor. How would you prioritise and manage your commitments?***

This question is testing your ability to cope under pressure. Avoid the pitfall of stating the order in which you choose to do your tasks, and leaving it at that – your reasoning is more important.

Use the following steps to answer the question:

- **Reiterate the tasks to be completed:** *"I have to work today, but need to take my child to hospital, as well as urgently complete a report."*
- **Identify the task with the greatest consequences:** *"The most serious task, in my opinion, is helping my sick child."*
- **Choose which task to complete first:** *"I will have to take my child to hospital today, and find a way to compensate for my other tasks."*
- **Identify the next most immediate task:** *"Next, I will deal with my work commitments."*
- **Set a game plan:** *"I will call work to explain that I cannot come into work today, due to my child being ill."*
- **Lessen the blow:** *"To make this as easy as possible, I will also call my colleagues and try to find someone to cover for me."*
- **Deal with the final task:** *"Finally, I will email my supervisor and explain the situation, and ask for an extension on my report."*

When it feels like you have too many commitments at once, communication is key. Communicate with the people who are relying on you so that they may make other arrangements.

Don't forget, however, that being a doctor comes with sincere responsibilities to care for your patients. It is important, therefore, that you seek some help in getting your duties covered from your colleagues.

8.8 *(MMI) A mother has come to the GP surgery with her 4-year-old daughter for a routine check-up. You check her immunisation record and advise that her daughter is due an 'MMR' vaccination. She refuses to have her daughter vaccinated because 'her nephew was immunised and now has autism'. She feels that this was a consequence of the MMR vaccine. Please respond to her concerns. The mother will be played by an actor in this station. You have 7 minutes.*

After introducing yourself and checking the patient's name and date of birth, you should approach this scenario with a basic structure, e.g.:

- **Enquire** – What is her main concern? What happened to her nephew? When did he have the vaccine? What does she know about the vaccine?
- **Empathise** – reassure her, acknowledge that she is concerned.
- **Explain** – benefits of immunisation, misconceptions about potential risks, current understanding of the vaccine's safety.
- **Explore** – What are her options? What action do you propose?
- **End** – briefly summarise, check for any questions.

Patients usually bring their own ideas, concerns and expectations to the consultation, which you should explore. As a doctor, you must always remember that you are treating patients and not just a set of signs and symptoms. A holistic approach should be adopted in every encounter to ensure you comprehensively cover the biological as well as the psychosocial aspects. Never dismiss a patient's concerns: this can be very discouraging.

Start by enquiring a little more about the origins of her concerns, e.g.: *"Please tell me a little more about your concerns..."*. Listen carefully to her response, making good eye contact and indicating that you are listening by using occasional brief verbal or non-verbal cues, such as *"Go on"*, *"OK"*, *"Right"*, *"Sure"*, or nodding occasionally to show that you understand.

Demonstrate to the interview panel that you can empathise with your patients, e.g.: *"Being a parent myself, I can understand your concerns..."*

Follow this up by dealing with any misconceptions she may have concerning the MMR vaccine. It is important to be honest when explaining benefits and risks to your patients, as this helps them to make a more informed decision. Explain that initial claims of a link between the vaccine and autism have since been disproven. Emphasise that there are greater risks in not immunising children, including infectious diseases and their potentially serious complications.

Now explore her options and propose suitable action. In this case, it is a good idea to allow her some time to properly absorb what has been discussed. Suggest that she discusses this with her partner. You may also want to provide her with additional information to take home to read. Finally, arrange for her to return in a few weeks to review any progress on the matter.

Conclude with a brief summary of what has been discussed and the suggestions you have both agreed on. Check that she has understood everything and ask if there are any questions.

8.9   **(MMI) You are a baker specialising in wedding cakes. A customer arrives expecting to collect her wedding cake. However, due to problems with the orders, the cake is not ready. You are responsible for explaining to the customer (played by an actor in this scenario), who has already paid a substantial deposit, that her cake won't be available for her wedding service later today.**

This scenario is designed to test your ability to deliver bad news. You should approach this scenario with a basic structure to your answer, e.g.:
- Introduce yourself and establish rapport
- Deliver the bad news
- Explain what went wrong and apologise
- Suggest what action will be taken to possibly resolve the problem.

Start by introducing yourself, checking who they are and establish rapport, e.g.: *"Good morning, can I just check your name please? I am Douglas, the head baker responsible for your wedding cake order. We spoke during your consultation earlier this year."*

Try not to keep your customer waiting for the bad news, as customers, like patients, generally prefer you to be honest and open with them regarding important issues. However, express your opening phrase carefully to prepare your customer for the bad news you are about to deliver, e.g.: *"Unfortunately, there is some bad news regarding your order..."*

Continue with an honest explanation, e.g.: *"We have been experiencing persistent problems with our IT system, which meant all current orders on our system were inaccessible. Regrettably, this included yours. I am very sorry about this."*

Allow the customer a few moments to absorb the bad news. Although the customer is likely to be angry, ensure that you remain calm in response to any criticism that may be directed at you. The importance of demonstrating empathy in such a situation cannot be overstated. Moreover, it will also help you to accept criticism more easily if you are able to consider the situation from her position.

You should also acknowledge that this is unacceptable for a professional service and take full responsibility for the situation. This will demonstrate your maturity and professionalism to the interview panel.

Most importantly, the customer will want to know what will be done to resolve this. You should therefore explain what immediate action you will undertake to help resolve the matter, e.g.: *"I will ask our local partner bakery to supply a replacement cake. Although this will not be to all your specifications, I will ensure that it does meet your dietary requirements. Needless to say, your deposit will be refunded immediately and you will not be charged for any services. You will also be issued with a £50 voucher as a goodwill gesture for the bad experience you have had."*

8.10 ***(MMI) Recently, your patient suffered an episode of loss of consciousness. According to the DVLA's instructions, you have advised her to suspend driving for 6 months. However, during a follow-up appointment it is clear that she has continued to drive. She assures you that she has been feeling much better lately and that she has not experienced any further episodes. Moreover, being a single parent, she explains that her two children rely on her to get to and from school, and that she needs the car to do the weekly shopping. Please discuss with the actor playing your patient what you will do, as her GP. You have 6 minutes.***

After introducing yourself and checking her name and date of birth, you should approach this scenario with a basic structure to your answer, e.g.: '**Enquire, empathise, explain, explore, end**'.

Start by **enquiring** about her driving: "*I understand that you are still driving at the moment...*". Try to deliver this in a natural, enquiring tone so that it doesn't sound too challenging. This will encourage her to be open with you.

Demonstrate **empathy** by acknowledging that driving is an important part of daily activities: "*I appreciate that this couldn't have come at a worse time, given the start of the school term.*"

However, **explain** that it is your duty to ensure she follows the DVLA's instructions, as it would be irresponsible and dangerous to let her continue driving if this could put her and others, including her children, at risk of harm. Try to explain this in a diplomatic way, e.g.: "*However, I must strongly advise that you refrain from driving for the remainder of the six months. I realise you feel you are well enough to drive as you have not experienced any further episodes, but these things are unpredictable, and it does not rule out the possibility of further episodes. I am sure you would agree this could have serious consequences if it happened whilst driving.*"

Hopefully, this will establish mutual agreement on the issue, which you can build on together by exploring possible ways of dealing with her circumstances. Remember that your role as a GP includes providing counsel to members of your community, who often seek your advice because they trust you.

As such, **explore** any practical solutions to her problem, e.g.: "*Is there anyone at all, perhaps a friend or relative, who could help you with the school run? Would it be possible to do the small shopping locally on foot, and maybe arrange to do the bigger shopping together with a friend or relative who drives?*"

Finally, bring the consultation to an **end** with a brief summary of what has been discussed. This gives your patient the opportunity to correct you or add anything else that may be relevant. It is a good idea to arrange another follow-up appointment for a few weeks' time to check how she is coping, both in terms of her health and with her practical situation.

8.11 *(MMI) You are the senior healthcare assistant on a hospital ward. Your role includes supervising and training new staff. After a busy shift, it has been brought to your attention that one of the new members (played by an actor in this scenario) was seen without appropriate personal protective equipment (PPE) during one of their duties. You have been asked to speak to her about the importance of using PPE and to discuss any problems. You have 7 minutes.*

This scenario tests your ability to demonstrate effective communication, teamwork and the initiative to overcome problems when working in a team.

After introducing yourself and checking the identity of who you are talking to, you can approach it with a similar structure to previous questions: '**Establish rapport, explain, explore, emphasise, end**'.

Start by **establishing rapport**. Be aware that, being new to the team, she may be nervous. Be friendly and smile to put her at ease. Try to convey a genuine interest in how she is settling in. It is often apparent to the interview panel when candidates have had previous experience in similar roles, as they are able to engage more naturally. This makes a very good first impression.

Now **explain** that you wanted to have a quick word with her about hospital policies. This will set the agenda for the meeting. You could mention that this is because she was seen not using PPE for some of her duties. However, deliver this in a diplomatic way so that it does not sound overly critical.

The actor portraying her may initially deny this, but you should not let this convince you, as the brief is very clear in its instructions. The interview panel will notice if you stray from these significantly, and you may risk giving a false impression that you would be easily influenced into glossing over such issues in a real situation. However, avoid being too challenging. Simply remind her that you are more than willing to go over anything she may not have understood during the induction.

Explore whether there was anything preventing her from using PPE as there may be a genuine reason, e.g. latex allergy, the appropriate size wasn't available, etc. This shows a willingness to consider things from her perspective. Mention that certain measures can be taken to accommodate any special requirements if this is necessary.

Emphasise the importance of using PPE. Educating her on the rationale for this is likely to encourage her compliance in future, e.g.: "*Wearing gloves and aprons in certain ward areas is part of our infection control and prevention policy, which helps to provide a safer environment for everyone.*"

Start bringing the meeting to an **end** by checking that she has understood everything and ask if she has any questions. Also, encourage her to ask for help if she has any problems. This will show her that you are approachable. Finally, thank her for coming to see you.

8.12 *(MMI) You are a first-year medical student. A friend of yours is struggling with the workload of the course and recently you have noticed them drinking more. You have agreed to go to lunch with them before a communication skills seminar that afternoon. Your friend wants to share a bottle of wine. Discuss whether this is appropriate behaviour with the actor, who will play the role of your friend in this scenario. You have 7 minutes to complete this station.*

This question will be an opportunity to show the examiner your basic communication skills and how you deal with a difficult situation.

When speaking with the friend:

- **Start by getting their view on this behaviour.** Use questions that allow your friend to speak openly and say what they want (termed 'open questioning'), ensuring they have the time to talk freely about the issue. You should try to ask questions in a non-judgmental way.
- **Explore your friend's thoughts on current drinking culture in general,** trying not to interrupt them excessively. You can then begin to focus on whether they think it is appropriate before medical school.
- **You may even want to direct your friend to further, more appropriate support** (such as their GP). This can be a difficult topic to broach with anyone, especially if this is your first attempt at doing so, but keeping calm, being empathetic, and staying focused will get you a large part of the way there.

The examiner for this station will want to see you are able to show empathy and understanding, whilst at the same time being logical, ethical, and rational in your conversation.

- If you have further time in this station (or any examiner present asks you questions following speaking to your 'friend'), **emphasise your need to escalate to a senior colleague or staff at the medical school if you feel it was appropriate.** Be ready to answer at what stage you would escalate to a senior.
- Professionalism will be an important part of your life as a medical student; thus, showing your appreciation for this topic will make you look knowledgeable and fully prepared for the start of medical student life.
- **If this was instead a hospital setting, patient safety is also an important priority.** A common question that can be asked is what to do if your registrar comes into work drunk whilst you are on your hospital clinical placement; an additional point to mention for a question such as this would be to ensure patient safety (e.g. ensuring no patients are treated by this doctor), the main focus of any practising healthcare professional in hospital.
- The examiner is not looking to catch you out, as often the most obvious answer at these stations tends to be the correct one!

8.13   **(MMI) You are a medical student shadowing a GP. During the consultation of a blind patient, neither the GP nor you obtains the patient's consent, i.e. asks if you can stay during the consultation. The patient only realises that you are present when he hears you asking the GP a question. He is quite upset. You are asked to discuss with an actor playing the role of the blind patient. You have 7 minutes.**

This scenario is testing your ability to communicate effectively with someone who is potentially very upset. You are expected to conduct yourself impartially and professionally in this sensitive situation.

You should follow these steps to deal with this scenario:

- **Introduce** yourself *"Hello, my name is Priya and I am a medical student."*
- Ensure that you have the correct person. Speak naturally and clearly; they are blind, but their hearing is not impaired.
- Find out if they want to have a discussion with you. Do not assume they have to; it is up to them. *"Would you like to talk to me about what happened earlier at your appointment?"*
- **Listen** patiently, giving the person a chance to explain their side of the story freely.
- Be polite and courteous.
- **Reflection**: empathise with the patient by stating the observed emotion – *"I can see you are quite upset".*
- **Legitimisation**: empathise with the patient – *"I can certainly understand why you are upset. You were not expecting or aware of the presence of another person in the consultation and no one asked for your permission. If I were in your position, I would probably feel the same way."*
- **Summarise** as you go along, in order to check your understanding with the patient.
- **Acknowledge, and apologise** for the mistake and make sure that the patient understands it would not have been done deliberately: *"We ask permission from every patient at the beginning of the consultation to check they are happy to have a student present. I understand this did not happen in your case and I unreservedly apologise for this oversight."*
- **Respect**: thank the patient for their time and for opening up to you – *"I appreciate the time you have taken to speak to me. It has really helped me understand your views and I can relay these to the GP, if you are happy with that."*
- **Support**: assure the patient that the situation will be discussed at the practice meeting and every step will be taken to ensure that a situation like this does not arise again.
- **Finish**: *"Is there anything else I can help you with?"*
- **Close** the conversation with *"Thank you, goodbye".*

All doctors are human beings and occasionally mistakes are made. It is important to acknowledge the patient's feelings, admit fault where there is one, provide an explanation as well as next steps to be taken to rectify the problem, and if they are still unhappy, tell them about the complaints procedure.

8.14 **(MMI) You share a house with several medical students. You notice lately one of your colleagues has been drinking a lot and staying in bed most of the day. He has started to miss lectures and is frequently borrowing notes from you. Yesterday he missed an important exam. You are concerned for his welfare and have decided to discuss with him. An actor will play the part of your housemate in this scenario. You have 7 minutes.**

This is a challenging scenario that is testing your ability to communicate effectively with someone who is in a very fragile state.

Your objective is to have a discussion with him and identify any problems. This is a chance for you to appear empathetic and communicate in a non-judgmental way.

Some suggestions (it might be worth mentioning some to the interviewer if they aren't possible to express in the scenario):
- Choose a private location where you can talk to your colleague without interruption.
- **Begin** by finding out how he has been finding his studies; perhaps he already recognises the problem: *"How are things going with your studies at the moment? Is everything OK?"*
- Convey your **concerns** for your colleague's wellbeing with specific statements such as
  - *"I have noticed that you haven't been yourself lately"*
  - *"I am worried about you and would like to help"*
  - *"Is there something that is bothering you?"*
- **Listen** to the response carefully and let him speak at his own pace.
- You must not sound patronising, otherwise he may be reluctant to speak to you.
- Probe whether the colleague is aware of the depth of the problem, e.g. by asking if he feels that his drinking is excessive and whether he has sought help for it.
- Remember to encourage him to seek help and offer to be there for him.

What not to do:
- Do not accuse or argue with him.
- Do not attempt to lecture; advice is OK if he seems open to it, but if in doubt, remain non-judgmental and listen.
- Do not give up; if he seems resistant or defensive, bring it up later.
- It may help to involve a trusted friend or family member, if you think they are more likely to help him open up.

You must remember your duty as a medical student to put patient safety first. It is likely that the medical school will already be aware of issues with the student if they are constantly missing teaching sessions. But if you know that the student is attending hospital/GP placements with hangovers, it is your responsibility to report this behaviour.

8.15 ***(MMI) You are a medical student on placement on a surgical ward. The F1 doctor is extremely busy, and asks you to take blood from several patients while she attends to a more urgent matter. Although you have taken blood before, you know that under your medical school rules, you are only able to take blood on the ward under supervision. Please discuss this with the F1, played by an actor. You have 7 minutes.***

Begin by acknowledging her request, and showing that you value the opportunity to practise your clinical skills.
"I really appreciate your trusting me with this task, and as you know, I am always happy to try to help out when the ward gets busy."

Establish an early rapport with the F1 doctor. However, when it comes to your response to her request, do not give an ambiguous answer. The rule is there to protect both patients and students from unsafe practice.

Explain this to the F1 doctor, ensuring you demonstrate to the examiner that you understand the reasons why the rule exists in the first place. Don't be tempted to agree to take the blood against the medical school rules, even if you are put under pressure to do so:
"However, I'm very sorry – I'm not able to take blood on this occasion, as the medical school rules explain that I can only do it under direct supervision."

Be empathetic – show that you see she is under a lot of stress and her request for help has not gone unheard: *"I see that you are extremely busy today – what else could I do to help?"*

If you are able to help with her urgent matter, find out how. It may be that your help frees up time for her to supervise you taking the blood from the patients: *"Could I be of any assistance while you deal with this urgent case?"*

You could offer to prepare the blood forms, collect the equipment, and run the blood down to the lab yourself once it is taken. There are many ways to be useful as a medical student on the ward: *"How about I prepare the equipment so we can quickly get to work taking the bloods after the urgent matter is resolved?"*

By giving alternatives to her suggestion, you are showing that you are adept at problem solving, and can think on your feet:
"I understand you don't have time to supervise me directly now; I will try to track down someone else to supervise me so I can do them as soon as possible."

Try to keep calm and maintain your position, even if your F1 doctor tries to persuade you otherwise. The station will show whether or not you can communicate effectively under pressure, and stand your ground even when pressed.

8.16 *(MMI) You are a GP. Your patient is a young woman who, although symptom-free, is worried about the prospect of cervical cancer. She notes several high-profile cases of cervical cancer being missed in young patients. She is 19 and screening begins at the age of 25. Cervical cancer occurs at a rate of 2.6 cases per 100 000 women under the age of 25. Please give your recommendation to your patient, and discuss her concerns with her. You have 7 minutes.*

Allow the patient time to voice her fears. Really listen to what she has to say, making a mental note of the main issues she raises so you can deal with each in turn when the time comes. Don't interrupt her or ask questions at this point.

When she has finished, begin by acknowledging her distress. Her fear is likely to be very real:
"I can see that you are really anxious about this issue. Thank you for being so honest with me today. Let's talk about each of the issues you have raised, and see if we can come to a decision about what to do next."

Clarify the incidence of cervical cancer in her age group. It may be useful to quote the numbers, but ensure you explain their significance, as it may not be immediately apparent to the patient.
"Cervical cancer occurs at a rate of 2.6 cases per 100 000 women in the under-25 age group. This means it is very rare – for every 100 000, less than 3 will have cervical cancer. For this reason, and the fact that young women may have abnormalities of the cervix that will resolve naturally over time, screening women under the age of 25 may do more harm than good. Therefore, I wouldn't recommend screening for a woman of your age."

This may not immediately settle her fears. Listen to her response, acknowledge her concerns, and answer the questions she has about the rationale for the screening age limit.

Give (appropriate) reassurance, especially since she is without symptoms, but don't give an absolute promise that she will never have gynaecological problems in the future; you cannot know this, and it is not likely to inspire confidence in your clinical opinion:
"I'm glad to hear you don't have any symptoms yourself. Tests for cervical cancer can be intrusive, and so doctors tend to use them only if they have good reason to suspect a patient may have the disease. You should, however, remain vigilant to any changes in your body."

You can use the opportunity to discuss the symptoms of cervical cancer (if you know them). The patient's fear may be reduced if you can give a good account of the symptoms to look out for, and why.

Use the opportunity to address her concerns sooner rather than later. Hopefully you have managed to allay some of her fears, but be prepared to discuss further if she is still not convinced by your recommendation:
"Is there anything you'd like to ask about the screening tests, so you are fully prepared to enter the screening programme when you turn 25?"

8.17 **(MMI) You are a supervisor at the research department of the university. You have spent several months conducting lab work with one of your PhD students, which is soon due to be submitted for publication in a leading journal. You have asked him to complete the write-up. However, with the deadline drawing closer, you have been told there has been little progress. You arrange a meeting with him to emphasise the urgency of the deadline, and to determine any barriers that may be hindering completion of the work. You have 7 minutes. An actor will play your PhD student.**

This scenario is designed to test your ability to manage and negotiate tasks with other members of your team, in this case your PhD student. You should approach this scenario with the same basic structure as used previously: '**Establish rapport, explain, enquire, emphasise**' but ensure you also offer suggestions and encouragement before **ending**.

Start with **establishing** rapport. Thank him for making it to the meeting as this conveys courtesy, e.g.: "*Good morning, thank you for coming to see me. Please take a seat.*"

Briefly **explain** the reason for meeting as this sets the agenda, e.g.: "*I thought it would be a good time to meet to discuss the write-up, because I was a bit concerned when you mentioned you have made little progress since the last draft.*"

In order to demonstrate effective teamwork, you must show the interview panel that you treat people fairly and are prepared to listen. You should therefore **enquire** about any specific problems that may have arisen, e.g.: "*I understand that your own research commitments have made it difficult to manage both tasks effectively. Is there anything else in particular that is demanding on your time?*" You don't know what's happening in their personal life – you must ensure they are not battling personal commitments too.

However, if there appear to be no personal problems it is your duty to **emphasise** the importance and urgency of this deadline, e.g.: "*As you will be aware, a great deal of resources have gone into this project.*"

Now **suggest** what action you will take to help with the situation. This way you are demonstrating a solution-focused approach, e.g.: "*Perhaps I can see if one of the others in the lab could carry out your lab work over the next few weeks whilst you complete the write-up. How does that sound?*"

Try to **end** with some encouraging words to lift his morale, e.g.: "*We have some great results and are very close to getting these published in a top journal with the help of your contribution.*" Finally, tell him to contact you if there are any more issues and extend your thanks again.

Chapter 9 | Ethics and decision making

9.1 *(T) Should abortion be made illegal?*

Abortion is a common issue brought up at interview due to the complex nature of the legal, ethical and even religious issues surrounding the topic.

It is important to know the law behind abortion, to state it for your interviewers and say as a practitioner you would abide by it. The 1967 Abortion Act legalised abortion, if conducted by registered medical practitioners, and facilitated the free provision of the service through the NHS. This Act originally made abortion legal when the mother was up to 28 weeks of gestation. The 1990 Human Fertilisation and Embryology Act was then introduced, which meant that abortion was no longer legal after 24 weeks, with exceptions being made for cases where there was a threat to the life of the mother, evidence of severe fetal abnormality or a risk of physical or mental injury to the woman.

A key distinction to be made is that in the eye of the law, an embryo or fetus has no rights. Instead they rest completely with the mother, an issue that is disagreed upon by religious organisations who believe that life starts at conception, rather than birth.

Doctors who are not in favour of abortion are not compelled to provide the service and can choose to abstain from the decision making process. They should, however, refer the patient to someone who will make a decision.

Once you have demonstrated your knowledge and understanding of the law, you should weigh up the ethical issues, focusing on the core ethical principles.

Pros of abortion	Cons of abortion
It may be in the **best interests** of the mother and child if bringing up a child will bring undue mental and physical stress to both mother and child.	For those who believe life begins at conception, abortion is analogous to murder. By facilitating abortion, it may devalue the sanctity of human life.
In order to protect the **autonomy** of the mother, she should be able to have the right to decide what happens to her own body.	Adoption is a healthy alternative. The mother does not have to look after an unwanted child, and the child grows in a home where he/she is wanted.
Many abortions occur in the first trimester, when the fetus cannot exist outside the mother's womb. Therefore, it cannot be considered a separate entity.	Abortion may cause physical harm to the mother, e.g. future miscarriages, ectopic pregnancies or pelvic inflammatory disease.
In the case of pregnancy secondary to rape, forcing a woman to carry on with the unwanted pregnancy may bring further psychological insult.	Abortion itself can cause intense psychological and emotional pain and suffering to the mother.

Once you have weighed up each side of the argument, you can state your own stance.

It is worth noting that the 1967 Abortion Act does not cover Northern Ireland, where the law surrounding abortion is different to the rest of the UK. For more information see *Question 16.8.*

9.2 (T) What do you think about assisted suicide and euthanasia?

Assisted suicide and euthanasia have consistently been topics of discussion at undergraduate interviews over the past decade. They have received widespread coverage across the media.

At the start of your answer, it is important to distinguish between assisted suicide and euthanasia. Euthanasia, also known as mercy killing, is the act of a **doctor ending** the life of a person with an incurable disease. Assisted suicide is the act of providing a person with the means to **end their own** life.

Knowing the law surrounding the issue helps to look at the situation objectively. Both euthanasia and assisted suicide are currently illegal in the UK. A few countries, e.g. Switzerland, have legalised assisted suicide.

The next step is to begin to discuss the pros and cons of the issue, some of which are summarised below. This should be focused on the core principles of medical ethics, highlighted in bold within the table below.

Pros of assisted suicide	Cons of assisted suicide
It enables **autonomy** for the patient, to be able to choose when and how they end their life.	The principle of **non-maleficence** states that a healthcare professional should not cause harm to the patient.
It may be in the **best interests** of the patient to end their life due to an unacceptable quality of life.	It risks the **trust** upon which the doctor–patient relationship is based.
It gives a method of relief when a person's quality of life is low or unacceptable to them.	Elderly patients may be coerced by their family to end their life due to the distress and inconvenience that their illness has on the family.
It provides a way to relieve extreme pain and distress in the final days of incurable suffering.	Risk of a 'slippery slope' whereby laws are created to enable terminally ill patients to end their life, but legislation may become relaxed to allow non-voluntary euthanasia.

At the end of the answer, you should make sure you balance the arguments and come up with a conclusion. Those who have considered and weighed up the issue often come across as strong candidates. Whatever your stance, be prepared to justify and defend it!

9.3   (T) Is human cloning ethically acceptable?

Most arguments are focused on the application of cloning for therapeutic reasons, whereby organs and tissues are generated to replace failing ones in another human. When initially answering this question, it is important to realise this can be achieved in two ways, each carrying slightly separate arguments.

The first is to insert genetic material into an empty oocyte and stimulate it to grow into an embryo and then implant it into a womb to grow as a fetus, subsequently to be born as a human. The second involves the artificial stimulation of stem cells to promote them to divide and create tissues.

It is important to note these arguments are very much theoretical, as human cloning has yet to be achieved. As always, this should be discussed with advantages and disadvantages balanced against each other, which are outlined below:

Advantages
- Cloning of failing organs can provide treatment to patients and remove the need for them to wait for donated organs.
- By using genetically identical organs, the patient avoids the risks of transplantation, including use of drugs that dampen the immune system.
- It offers another alternative for couples unable to conceive and for whom IVF did not work.

Disadvantages
- Some who believe that life starts as an embryo, do not agree with the extent that embryos are destroyed whilst attempting to clone, and liken it to murder.
- In addition, some religious groups may claim that the technology is replacing the role of God in human creation.
- There is the potential for abuse of the technology where generations of humans are born simply to harvest tissues from.

Finally, you may wish to discuss recent technology involving stem cell replication, whereby the possibility exists of rejuvenating damaged organs. In this scenario, healthy stem cells are implanted in damaged tissues (for example, after a heart attack) and allow regeneration of healthy tissue. This is applicable to many degenerative diseases such as Parkinson's, arthritis and Alzheimer's disease. This does not seem to undergo the same ethical debate that therapeutic cloning does and therefore may prove to be a viable option in the future.

Conclude your answer by stating that the ethical debate behind cloning is varied depending upon which technique is being referred to. Make sure your argument is balanced so you can discuss any point in more detail.

9.4 (T) If you were the Health Secretary, and had an extra £1 million, what single new intervention or policy would you put in place?

This question is very open ended, and another common theme within medical school interviews. The interviewers will be looking to see whether you understand what the current health problems are within society and if you can bring forward an appropriate potential plan to solve them. It tests your knowledge and understanding of multiple issues including epidemiology, public health and health economics.

Firstly, you should identify an issue that either affects a large proportion of the population, or that is currently underfunded.

33% of all mortality in the UK is due to cardiovascular disease, comprising heart disease (23%) and stroke (10%). Cancer forms the next biggest chunk, representing 30% of all deaths. Other increasingly important problems that can be discussed are obesity (which links to heart disease), mental health (which is under-recognised and underfunded) and social care (which prevents patients from becoming ill and requiring hospital admissions).

In the case of cardiovascular disease, you have the opportunity to show off a little medical knowledge as well, by stating risk factors. These include smoking, obesity, high blood pressure and cholesterol levels, all of which could be potential targets for your funding. Social care gives you the opportunity to discuss primary health care, and also shows your understanding of the working of a multidisciplinary team outside of hospital care, such as the role of general practitioners, carers, occupational/physical therapists, district nurses and social workers.

The next step is to tackle the problem and this is where 'health economics' comes into the equation. Your solution needs to be viable, affordable, and provide the largest benefit to the population. Here, the 'prevention paradox' is a key epidemiological principle to adhere to. In a situation where large numbers of people are exposed to a small risk, more disease will be generated than when a few individuals are exposed to a large risk. Conversely, however, if a small benefit is applied to a large number of people, the benefit will also be large.

The topic you pick will mostly be determined by which one you have the most knowledge about and can discuss in detail. Taking the example of social care, this may mean increasing funding for social care, such that elderly patients can receive support from their carers and district nurses in their own home. If this is effective, it will improve the health of these patients and prevent hospital admissions, which in turn will free hospital beds for acutely unwell patients and save the NHS money overall.

TOP TIP The interviewer may challenge your idea. Don't be shocked; the interviewer is trying to see not only whether you can defend your plans, but also whether you have the insight to acknowledge any limitations in your plans.

9.5   (T) Children born severely prematurely (under 22 weeks) have a very low chance of survival. Therefore, do you think it is ethically acceptable to deny them medical care?

Neonatal ethics is a complex topic, affected greatly by the emotion of parents and relatives. Whilst medical technology has dramatically reduced mortality (i.e. death) rates for newborn children, their quality of life remains a big issue.

The question posed here brings together discussions based on quality of life and resource allocation, additionally giving the candidate a chance to demonstrate empathy towards a difficult decision that must be faced by clinicians and parents.

To enable you to answer this question, you should first know the guidance that is available to doctors faced with this situation. The Nuffield Council on Bioethics has produced guidance on the issue and it has suggested that babies of less than 22 weeks' gestation should not receive resuscitation, those of 22–23 weeks' gestation should also not receive resuscitation unless asked for by the parents, the parents of babies of 23–24 weeks' gestation should be given the option of treatment and at 24–25 weeks' gestation intensive care should be given unless both parents and medical staff agree otherwise. For those greater than 25 weeks, intensive care should be given.

A child born before 22 weeks has only a 1% chance of surviving beyond hospital. With such low survival rates, treatment may only prolong suffering for both the child and parents. Supporters of this view may argue that if life consists purely of pain and suffering then inflicting this is simply inhumane.

Of those that do survive, many leave hospital suffering with severe disabilities, which may impact on the patient and the family, who will be put through extra physical and psychological burden as a result. However, opponents will argue that there are plenty of examples of disabled individuals who have led fulfilling lives.

Finally, neonatal intensive care comes at a high price. Therefore, with such low success rates at 22 weeks, should these resources be spent elsewhere? Why should we deny some patients expensive cancer drugs but provide futile treatment for neonates? Those who disagree with this point of view may argue that it is immoral to place a value on a human life. Furthermore, how does one calculate and value it?

When you conclude your arguments, it is important to let the examiners know you recognise this is a complex situation with multiple aspects that must be considered before making a decision. If faced with this scenario, you should state that this is a decision you would make after seeking the advice of seniors and the multidisciplinary team. You should state your own views on the issue, but make sure that you have brought up opposing arguments over the course of your answer to ensure that your position can be justified and defended.

9.6 (MMI) You are in charge of the liver transplantation unit. You have the choice of giving a transplant to a 70-year-old alcoholic or a 27-year-old single mother with auto-immune hepatitis. Who would you give the transplant to? You have 2 minutes to gather your thoughts and then 6 minutes to present to the interviewer.

When answering this question, there are some basic facts about transplantation that you should be aware of and point out to the interviewer. Both patients have a need for the transplant, but before they can receive it, there are some considerations. Both patients require genetically compatible organs in order to receive a transplant, and must be medically fit to tolerate the operation. If either of the patients doesn't fulfil these criteria, the other should be considered to receive the transplant.

Once you have demonstrated a basic understanding of your knowledge of the topic, start to discuss the ethical issues. The major issue here is of one patient who has a lifestyle-inflicted disease, whilst the other is a result of an uncontrollable process of inheritance. The main issues behind this case of distributive justice are:

- As the mother's disease is no fault of her own, she should receive priority over a patient who has chosen a lifestyle with the knowledge of the potential harm it would cause.
- The alcoholic patient may continue to drink in the future, which would damage the transplanted liver.
- Likewise, if the underlying disease for the mother is not controlled, the same disease may then proceed to destroy the transplanted liver.

The next issue is age:

- The alcoholic patient is already 70 years old. They may not have many years of healthy life left, and if they pass away in a few years, the potential life of the transplant is wasted.
- Conversely, the mother is young and may even 'outlive' the transplant, making full use of it.

Finally, the issue of dependants:

- The mother has dependent children, meaning that if she does not receive the transplant her children risk being orphaned.
- The elderly alcoholic patient is unlikely to have dependants, yet still may have a family who would be affected by a decline in his health.

When summarising you should point out that the complexities of this case mean you would be uncomfortable in making this decision by yourself, both now and in the future as a clinician. At this point, you should state you would enlist the help of the multidisciplinary team, including hepatologists, transplant surgeons, specialist nurses and patient advocates.

9.7 (T) Would you report a senior doctor with whom you were working if you thought that they were practising in a way that was endangering patients?

This question is assessing the methods you would use to deal with a challenging situation but one that affects patient care. It also is gauging your professionalism.

The best way to answer this question is to break it down into steps. This gives you time to think and allows the interviewer to follow your thoughts.

Step one – show rational thought, and do not jump to a direct answer:
"Firstly I would have to justify why I thought that the senior doctor was endangering patients."

Step two – discuss the methods that you could use to justify your conclusion:
- Be humble enough to ask the doctor to explain some of the decisions they have made. It may not be incompetence if they made a decision based on information that you do not yet know about. This may potentially be the case until you have years of experience.
- Check your own medical knowledge; for example, if the doctor was making incorrect diagnoses, or he had inadequate clinical skills make sure you understand the area.
- Talk to a colleague about the problem, maintaining the senior doctor's anonymity; you may be able to understand the situation better once you have discussed it.

Step three – continue to explain what you would do if the doctor was in fact incompetent:
"Ultimately patients are of paramount importance and therefore, if their care was at risk it would be appropriate to speak to the senior doctor, or if this wasn't easy to do (are they not approachable?) to ask for help and advice from another senior doctor."

9.8 (T) If you had a place at medical school would you step down so that a friend who did not get a place could have yours? Please justify your answer.

One of the most important attributes of a doctor is empathy, and it is key to demonstrate this trait during an interview. Although this question requires you to acknowledge the feelings of your friend it is also expecting you to demonstrate confidence in yourself as the best candidate for the place on the course.

You could begin answering with a statement such as:
"Although I would be disappointed for my friend I believe that I would make a good doctor and so I would not step down so that my friend could have my place."

Next you need to justify this decision. You can do so by explaining why you should take the place, whilst considering ways of being considerate to your friend. The following types of statement may help you do that:
"I would discuss with the friend about why they think that they did not get a place at medical school, in the hope of strengthening their application for the following year."

"I am confident that I want to pursue a career in medicine and if I was to turn down a place at medical school I may not have another opportunity."

"The medical school application process is rigorous and I have faith in it to choose the most appropriate people to be doctors. Therefore, despite this question being a hypothetical one, respecting the system would be the right thing to do."

9.9 (T) What are the four principles of ethics in medicine, and why do you think it is important to adhere to them?

The four basic principles of biomedical ethics are:

1. **Respect for autonomy**

   Autonomy describes the fundamental tenet that doctors and healthcare professionals must at all times respect the decision-making capability of the competent patient who has full capacity. The patient must be respected and given all the necessary information, and the doctor should share this to allow the patient to make a fully informed decision about their treatment. Respecting patients' autonomy extends also to scenarios where a competent patient makes a decision against medical advice, however hard that may be for the doctor to understand. This is important because it respects the patient's wishes and preserves their right to make decisions over their own body and life.

2. **Beneficence**

   This refers to the rule that doctors must always act in the best interest of their patients. This enables patients to maintain trust in their doctor.

3. **Non-maleficence**

   This is a popular phrase in medicine, meaning 'Do no harm'. It refers to the rule that the doctor must always seek to minimise harm to the patient, and must first and foremost act in a way that prevents further damage to a patient's health. For example, if a patient is offered a treatment which the doctor is not sure will benefit the patient, the doctor must also verify that the treatment doesn't harm the patient in any way as well. This is important again because of the sanctity of the patient's trust in doctors.

4. **Justice**

   This refers to the rule that doctors and healthcare practitioners should act in a way that is fair to all patients, and must always act with moral resolution.

These are all important because healthcare is very personal and patients are potentially quite vulnerable. Doctors must therefore be ethical and trusted in order to treat people in their time of need.

9.10   *(MMI) An 86-year-old Asian lady (who does not speak English) is in the hospital. Your investigations show that she has terminal cancer. Her daughter does not want you to tell her mother, as this would be 'too distressing for her'. Please discuss how you are going to proceed with the daughter, who will be played by an actor. You have 7 minutes.*

This question is seeking to know if you understand the different issues within the scenario and if you can come up with a way to deal with them in a logical and ethical way.

First of all, you need to let the interviewers know that you understand the extent of the situation.

This patient has a terminal condition and needs to be fully informed of this, irrespective of the family's wishes.

You should first ask the daughter what concerns her about her mother finding out. Does she not normally cope well with bad news? There might be more to the story and it is important that you build a rapport with the daughter. You should be empathetic to the daughter and explain to her why her mother needs to know.

Begin with a sentence that addresses the fact that it is a horrible situation to be in.
"I can see this is a very difficult time for you and your family; however, it is important that your mother knows what is going on. As a doctor I'm afraid we are duty bound to explain honestly to your mother about what is happening."

Explain that you still care for her mother:
"This is a very challenging time and I give you my assurance that I will explain this in the gentlest way possible."

It would be really useful to read the GMC's *Good Medical Practice* (2013) to get a better idea of how to deal with difficult situations, as the GMC has guidelines to many common scenarios.

Another issue in this scenario is the fact the patient does not speak English. You should request an interpreter as they are trained to translate medical terminology and are professionals. There are many disadvantages to using family members as interpreters, especially in this scenario as the family could withhold information.

9.11 (T) Junior doctors have recently gone on strike. Do you think it is ethical for doctors to strike?

It is important to be familiar with the issues surrounding the junior doctors' strikes. Read more about the issues surrounding the junior doctor contract dispute in *Question 14.17*.

Background

It is relatively rare for doctors to strike, and the current industrial action garnered overwhelming support from balloted junior doctor members of the British Medical Association, 99% of whom voted for strike action and 98% of whom even supported a full walkout. A number of strikes, starting with junior doctors providing emergency care only, commenced in December 2015 and continued into 2016. This was the first such strike by junior doctors since November 1975.

As with any ethics question it is important to display both sides of the argument, but also be prepared to answer the personal question, *"If you were meant to be at work on a strike day, what would you do?"*

Against doctors striking:

- Some may argue that those employed in the public sector providing an essential service should not be able to strike, similar to police officers in the UK.
- Patients may come to harm if medical staff are not at work, especially if there is a full walkout.
- Even without a full walkout, non-emergency tests and operations were cancelled, e.g. potentially delaying cancer diagnosis and treatment.

In favour of doctors striking:

- Evidence from strikes in other international healthcare systems has shown that patients are not adversely affected by junior doctor strikes (and in fact may even receive *better* care, since consultants cancel their administration, research or teaching commitments and provide the direct patient care in place of the junior doctors).
- Medical doctors are under tremendous pressure, and the nature of the job brings high rates of burnout and difficulty in maintaining a work/life balance. Protection of human rights and being able to strike are thus important defence strategies.
- Doctors have a professional and ethical duty to challenge (e.g. by strike action, if they can ensure patients do not come to harm) other stakeholders on decisions such as contracts where patient safety may be compromised.

9.12 **(MMI) You are in the operating theatre as a medical student and realise that a consultant is about to amputate the wrong leg. In this scenario a mock operating theatre will be set up and your interviewer will play the role of the consultant. Please interact with them, knowing that they are about to amputate the wrong leg. There will be other 'members of staff' in the room too, including a scrub nurse, an anaesthetist and a senior nurse. The X-ray is on the computer screen. You have 7 minutes.**

This is a difficult situation, because you are required to correct a senior and more experienced professional. This station will test your communication skills and your ability to act quickly and confidently in a critical situation. It is important that you do speak up if you notice a mistake of this magnitude about to take place. If you were to query the consultant and you were mistaken, you may feel a little embarrassed; however, if you were not mistaken and did not speak up then the patient losing a healthy leg would be a far worse outcome.

You have to be clear and accurate.
- **Introduce yourself** (in theatre, everyone normally introduces themselves before the operation begins to allow everyone to feel they have a voice in case of this very scenario; however, it is possible that if the consultant is focused on the operation ahead he may not remember specifically who you are): *"Hello Mr Smith, I am John Jones, the medical student observing your theatre list today."*
- **Explain very clearly the mistake that you have observed:** *"I was reading the notes for this patient, and I have noticed that it is his left leg that was identified for amputation. However, here the right leg has been prepared for surgery. I think there may have been a mistake."*

The good interviewer may take this a step further – don't be put off by this. They may simply be giving you the chance to flourish. They may ask something like:
"The consultant tells you to keep quiet – you are just a medical student. What do you do?" (This is unlikely to happen in real life in this scenario but in an interview it is a question that can be used to discriminate between a good candidate and an excellent one.)

This is urgent. You work as part of the team and if you are not being listened to because you are junior then you need some senior help. You may want to:
- Discuss immediately with the anaesthetist looking after the patient – they may also be a consultant and be able to help intervene.
- Make sure the X-rays are on the computer screen and highlight them to the consultant.
- Ask for urgent help from one of the senior theatre nurses – they may also be able to speak to the surgeon with some authority.

9.13 *(T) You are working as a GP. A 14-year-old female patient tells you that she is pregnant. What do you do? Would it be right to inform the girl's parents about the pregnancy against her wishes? What about informing other health or social care professionals?*

This is quite a complex scenario but it is not uncommon for girls under the age of 16 to require sexual health services and support.

There are a number of conflicting medical principles that require consideration in this scenario: confidentiality, consent and safeguarding children. You will not be expected to have detailed knowledge of these principles but you should be able to form an answer that takes into account the girl's wishes and her safety.

There are some salient points that you need to take into consideration:

- The 14-year-old girl has approached you in confidence about her pregnancy. You are duty bound to maintain her confidentiality unless you believe that her right to privacy is outweighed by a risk to her safety. This may be the case if she has a much older partner or if you believe that she was coerced into sexual activity. This may not require the involvement of her parents but might mean a discussion with another doctor or with social services.
- Some 14-year-old girls would have sufficient understanding of their situation to make their own choices regarding treatment. If you feel she doesn't, however, you may also be justified in discussing the case with her parents or carers.
- If she is a competent 14-year-old girl you should encourage her to talk to her parents or another responsible adult such as a school nurse, youth worker or relative.
- The situation becomes much more complex if the girl tells you the sexual partner was much older. This introduces a legal aspect of child sexual abuse. In this scenario it would be advisable to seek some senior advice as to what to do, from a senior partner in the GP practice, your medical defence union and the team that deals with child abuse (often called the 'safeguarding team').

9.14 *(MMI) You have finished school and are enjoying the summer before you begin university. You are at a party and notice one of your friends, who you know to be pregnant, consuming a large amount of alcohol. Explain how you would handle this situation. You have 7 minutes to complete this station.*

This challenging scenario is designed to assess your ability to recognise the ethical issues at play, as well as your ability to communicate effectively and empathetically with one of your peers. This is not designed to assess what you know about the harmful effects of alcohol on the unborn child, and candidates who treat it like that will not score highly. More importantly, it is vital that you can show you are an empathetic person.

This scenario should be approached as follows:
- Initially, you should make the point that you wouldn't speak to your friend regarding this very sensitive issue while they are drunk: this would be inappropriate. Rather, it would be better to wait until the next day, when you should make arrangements to speak to your friend in person.
- To initiate the conversation, it would be best to ask in very general terms how your friend is getting on: *"How have things been with you recently?"* This is a non-threatening way of opening the conversation, and you should allow your friend plenty of time to talk without interrupting them (GPs talk about the 'golden minute' at the start of a consultation to allow the patient to describe the problem in their own terms).
- Following this introduction, and depending on how your friend responds, it may be appropriate to ask about her feelings regarding the pregnancy.
- You will not perform well in this station if you enter into a strident rant about the dangers of alcohol to your friend's unborn child. A more considered way of approaching it would be to find out if there is anything in particular that your friend is struggling with, and whether there is anything you can do to help her: *"Is there anything troubling you at the moment? I was wondering if you needed help with anything at all?"*
- However, it would be wrong to ignore the issue of the alcohol consumption completely. It should be addressed sensitively *"I was wondering if you had thought much about drinking alcohol during pregnancy?"*
- After asking this question, it would be worth gently mentioning that alcohol has been known to cause damage to children in the womb, and that your friend should think about cutting down or eliminating her alcohol intake.
- Finish the conversation by saying that your friend can speak to you at any time with any problems she has, and if she has any questions about her pregnancy in particular she should contact her GP.

9.15 **(MMI) You begin your first job as a junior doctor, and are lucky enough to be placed on the same ward as your best friend from medical school. However, over the past few weeks you have noticed that they have become increasingly distant and uninterested in their work. One day, you notice them taking a tablet of a morphine-based painkiller from the drugs cabinet and swallowing it. Please discuss with your best friend, who will be played by an actor. You have 7 minutes to complete this station.**

First and foremost, this scenario gives you the chance to demonstrate that patient safety is paramount. It should be at the forefront of your mind in everything you do as a doctor. However, it is complicated by the fact that your best friend is involved, creating a clear conflict of interest. The candidate who approaches this sensitively, with involvement of the correct people and who ensures patient safety is maintained, will score highly.

- Begin by asking your friend/colleague to speak to you in private, e.g. in a ward side room or office. It would be highly inappropriate and potentially distressing to have this conversation within earshot of patients.

- It is best not to adopt an accusatory, authoritative manner when dealing with situations such as this, and you should begin by asking your friend/colleague if they have taken anything they shouldn't have. They may deny this, but you should still begin by asking them.

- Inform them of the risk to patient safety, and tell them you think they shouldn't continue working today: *"I saw you take some morphine from the drugs cabinet and swallow it, so you really shouldn't be looking after any patients today. I think you should call a taxi and go home".*

- Suggesting calling a taxi to take them home shows that you are concerned for the safety of your friend/colleague as well (would they be fit to drive after taking some morphine?).

- It may be worth suggesting that you would ensure the patients your friend has treated this morning are all fine and have had safe decisions made for them – especially if the doctor may have been under the influence of prescription drugs.

- As always in situations such as this, it is important to explore any issues that may be underlying the change in behaviour. Have they been struggling with the workload? Have they seen things at work that have upset them? Do they have financial concerns? Have they been having issues in their personal lives?

- Inform your friend/colleague that you are going to have to tell the consultant in charge of the ward what you saw, because of the risk to patient safety (mentioning these two words more than once will do your answer no harm at all) and that because you are their friend, you aren't best placed to make decisions in this case.

- Thank your friend for speaking to you and make a point of saying that you would speak personally to your supervising consultant as soon as possible about this issue.

9.16 **(MMI) You are a consultant surgeon. A few days ago, you performed what was supposed to be a straightforward surgical procedure on an elderly gentleman. Due to an error during the operation, the patient lost more blood than was anticipated, and the patient unfortunately died last night. You are about to have a meeting with the patient's son, a barrister, who will be played by an actor. Answer any questions he may have. You have 7 minutes to complete this station.**

This would be a highly emotive interaction, and you should demonstrate yourself to be aware of this by being sensitive and understanding:

- Introduce yourself according to the description of the situation. Mention to the examiner that you would like to have the discussion in a quiet room, free from any possible interruptions (e.g. your mobile phone).
- Establish that you are speaking to the correct person. *"May I just check who I am speaking to, to avoid any confusion?"*
- Once you have confirmed that it is the patient's son that you are speaking to, assess his understanding of the scenario so far, so you don't spend time labouring a point he is already aware of.
- You should offer an apology. This is not an admission of guilt or responsibility! It is a way of demonstrating sympathy and building a rapport with the patient's son.
- It is important to be honest, and not to try to cover up what happened. *"I am very sorry for what happened with your father. He died as a result of an error during the operation that led to him losing more blood than anticipated. We did all we could to save his life following this, but we were unable to do so".*
- Explain to the son that because he died soon after an operation, his father must go for a post-mortem examination before his funeral can take place. *"Legally, because of the circumstances in which your father died, a post-mortem examination must take place. I am aware this could make things even more difficult for your family, but this process helps us to learn, to ensure things like this don't happen again".*
- Assure the son that his father's death has been taken very seriously by the whole team involved, and that his case will be discussed at the Morbidity and Mortality meeting for the surgical unit (these are regular meetings where all the staff within a unit gather to discuss patients that have come to harm or have died in their unit, in an effort to improve patient safety. Any interviewer would be very impressed if you were able to reference a process like this at such an early stage in your career).
- Ask the son if he has any questions he wants to ask you. Tell him that he can contact you at any time to discuss things again.
- Thank the son for meeting with you and offer your sympathies once again.

N.B. The fact that the son is a barrister should make no difference to how you approach this scenario!

9.17 **(MMI) You are currently in sixth form and an overweight friend of yours knows you want to do medicine. They have been struggling with their weight for a few years now and have been bullied regularly since starting at the school. They ask for your advice about how they could lose some weight. Please discuss with your friend, who will be played by an actor. You have 7 minutes to complete this station.**

This station will be primarily focused on your communication skills, empathy, and decision making. You may have already been through a similar scenario whilst at sixth form and it is a difficult situation to be put in. In this station, being a good communicator is key, so ensure you give your friend plenty of time to speak about everything that is worrying them.

You may want to approach this station by finding out more details about what has been going on recently, with both their weight and being bullied. As is widely publicised, being bullied can cause an individual great emotional damage, so (depending on the station) talking not only about the weight problems but also the underlying causative issues may be appropriate. Be open in your questioning and do not be judgmental, simply smiling and being pleasant can go a long way!

When discussing the weight loss, this is another opportunity to show your communication skills to the examiner. Work through any discussion with a systematic approach:
- **Start by asking them what they have tried in the past**. If your friend has not tried any ways to lose weight, then you can advise simple measures to do so, such as exercise or healthy eating.
  - Do not feel you have to come up with an original answer. Keeping it simple and relevant is more important.
- **Next, perhaps ask them what they are currently trying or currently thinking about**. Depending on the station, it may be that your friend may want to try something more invasive, such as gastric band surgery.
  - If you feel you are being pushed during the station, that is usually a good sign; the interviewer is likely to be trying to see the extent of your communication skills and if you can cope with a more stressful situation.
- **Remember to reassure your friend** and offer the opportunity for further support in the future. This is likely to be a very difficult time for them, so knowing they have the support of a friend will help them immensely.

Overall, there is no right or wrong answer for this question, and the above is simply a suggested structure. Most importantly, show empathy and good listening skills.

9.18   *(MMI) You are a GP in a large practice, in which you look after three generations of the same family. A daughter of this family has come to your surgery quite angry because her father came to see you a while ago feeling unwell and you did not take any major action at the time, as you believed no clinical evidence supported any action being taken. He was later admitted to hospital and sadly died. Please discuss with the daughter, who will be played by an actor. You have 7 minutes to complete this station.*

An examiner at this station will want to see you showing some key skills of a potential doctor, including your listening skills and empathy. This scenario may be common for many general practitioners. It requires sensitivity towards the family member in providing the exact details of the event and ensuring a continued relationship with that particular family.

When approaching this station, be structured, honest and empathetic.
- **Start by listening to the daughter.** Staying silent and understanding the daughter's complaints will benefit you early in the consultation, as you can learn a lot of information about what is troubling her. Ensuring you get all these details will allow you to provide a much better answer in response. Do not underestimate the importance of staying quiet and just listening to the daughter! Use body language to demonstrate you are listening – occasionally nodding and maintaining eye contact (but not staring!).
- **Offer an apology early on if you have done something wrong!** As mentioned elsewhere, you can also use the phrase, *"I'm sorry to hear about this"* or *"I'm sorry for what has happened to your father."*
- **If and when appropriate, explain the reasoning behind your clinical decision.** Read the opening statement given to you before the interview carefully, as this will form the bulk of your discussion. If true, the mainstay of your answer will be that you were confident in the decisions you made and there were no indications at the original consultation to suggest any concern with her father.
  A significant part of this station will revolve around your listening skills, so listen to any further concerns the daughter has and address them as you see fit (do not worry about getting the medical details exactly right; the examiner at this station will want to see your communication skills, not your scientific knowledge).
- **To conclude, depending on the specifics for the station, you may be required to offer further solutions to the daughter.** This may involve arranging another appointment to see you again or even offering grief counselling. Addressing all the patient's concerns will keep their trust.
  Keep calm, show empathy to the daughter, and be structured in your responses.

9.19 **(MMI) You are doing work experience at a needle exchange programme. The friend of a service user tells you that he simply rinses needles and uses them again, and shares them with his friends. He and his friends are in good health; therefore he thinks the needle exchange is a waste of time. Please explain to the friend, who will be played by an actor, why you think he might be better off using the service. You have 7 minutes.**

Introduce yourself to the service user's friend, and briefly explain your role.

"My name is Faisal. I'm doing work experience here at the programme. As you know, we provide clean needles to anyone who needs them, as we are trying to minimise the risk of diseases spreading by the sharing of needles. Thanks for coming to chat with me – do you mind if we discuss what you just told me?"

This person is engaging in risky behaviour, both in the abuse of illicit drugs and in the sharing of needles. They need your support and guidance, rather than your condemnation. There is a stigma attached to being an intravenous drug user – do not be tempted to reinforce this by being judgmental or overly critical.

"You have told me that you have been reusing your needles and sharing them with friends. Do you know the reasons why we discourage this practice?"

Just like any other explanation, assess the extent of their knowledge before you proceed, adapting language and content accordingly.

"Some potentially life-threatening diseases, such as hepatitis B and C, and HIV, can be contracted through contamination of shared needles with body fluids such as blood. By sharing needles, however clean they may seem, you will put yourself and the people around you at risk of becoming ill."

You may encounter a combative attitude, or provocation (he has already shown he is scornful of the programme, considering it a 'waste of time'). Although you must ensure he is made fully aware of the potential harm that recklessness with needles may cause, don't allow yourself to be anything other than calm and sympathetic.

"We recommend you use clean needles for your own safety, but also for the protection of those around you. I know you must care for your friends, so it's in all your interests to return your needles to the programme and receive a fresh batch."

Appeal to his compassionate side. It is critical that he is made aware of the risks to himself and others, as you would be doing him and other users a disservice if you didn't emphasise this point.

"Remember, there are always people here to support you – whether that's in helping you maintain safe practice at home, or if you need help to stop using altogether. Thanks for talking to me today."

Chapter 10 | Abstract questions

10.1 **(T) If you were in a burning house and could only take one item with you, what would you take, and why?**

This is an opportunity to appear thoughtful and considerate. It also allows you to express your personality and to appear empathetic.

An example:
"This is a challenging question and until I would be in that circumstance it may be difficult to answer [shows thoughtfulness] but one of the things I am most passionate about is..."

Now: What are you passionate about? Or, what couldn't you live without? You can pick most things – within reason – so long as you can justify it and so long as it doesn't sound too clichéd.
"I would take my photo album. This is because it contains pictures of all of my closest relatives and friends. I am a firm believer that health is about mental and physical wellbeing. Because these people have had such a profound impact on my life I would be distraught not to have their memories with me.

I know I can get food and water elsewhere, but it is difficult to recover emotional loss."

Now link it to medicine...
"Without their support I would find it difficult to be here applying for medicine today. This realisation will hopefully make me a better doctor because it will provide me with the empathy and compassion to treat people as human beings.

It will help me to communicate with both patients and their families."

10.2 *(MMI) You are meeting a charity who would like to invest in improving global health. You have been asked to give a presentation to two of their directors (played by your interviewers) that will convince them to invest in your idea for global health. You may use the flip chart provided. You have 5 minutes to prepare and 5 minutes to give your presentation.*

Presenting and public speaking is a key skill for doctors. This is a chance to be an individual in the interview and stand out. Your plan to improve global health must be suitably detailed, realistic and preferably of benefit to a large number of people. Choose a recent issue you would like to help resolve.

Use the flip chart to draw colourful diagrams and outline key points. Don't just read out your points but talk around them. Remember to introduce yourself and what you intend to cover in your presentation at the start. Thank the audience/invite questions at the end.

Introduce your global health initiative:
"Thank you for allowing me to discuss my proposals today. I would like to concentrate on an area of the world where there is poor access to healthcare. The health issue I feel strongly about is childhood vaccinations. Low-income countries are associated with a high infant mortality rate and the lack of childhood vaccinations is a major contributing factor. A suitable disease to vaccinate children against would be diphtheria in a location such as sub-Saharan Africa. I would vaccinate children aged under 5."

Explain your choice:
"Vaccination programmes offer excellent efficacy with high impact, as a large population can be protected from a disease at a relatively low initial cost and with little follow-up."

Now talk about potential barriers and how you will overcome them:
"Mistrust and lack of awareness are major barriers to the success of a foreign vaccination initiative so I would prefer to fund local charities and local institutions to organise and give the vaccinations. The population cover for diphtheria will need to be as high as 95% and rural areas will be difficult to travel to. I expect this programme to be completed within 5 years per country in sub-Saharan Africa, but the speed of delivery mainly depends on how much money is available."

Other global health initiatives:
- Access to safe water
- Combating child malnutrition
- Access to improved healthcare for refugees
- Reducing maternal death rates
- Combating HIV/AIDS epidemic.

10.3 **(MMI) In your current attachment your fellow medical student has been shouted at by a patient. They ask if you have ever been shouted at and how you dealt with it. Please also relate this experience to your colleague's situation. You have 7 minutes. The assessor will play your fellow medical student.**

Here, your emotional intelligence is being tested. How you cope with conflict and how you operate in a pressured environment are all key issues. There is no single correct answer to this but there are wrong ones. Avoid describing reactions that involve negative stress-releasing behaviour, including causing harm or any form of violence! Be honest in your answer and relate a true-life experience.

- **Set the scene:**

"It is difficult to describe one reaction, as each situation is individual. It may depend on my setting and on who is shouting at me. On occasions when I have been shouted at, I have always sought to respond in a calm manner and to solve the problem if possible. For example, last month in a homeless soup kitchen, where I volunteer to hand out soup, I was accosted by a woman who demanded more soup. The centre is very busy so we have strict guidelines to only give one portion of soup per person. This lady wanted to take two portions and when I refused, she began shouting and verbally abusing me."

- **How you felt:**

"Initially I felt a little shocked and threatened. I also felt frustrated because I was trying to help the centre and the people who use it. I reminded myself of the lady's unfortunate situation and began to understand her anger. I felt empathetic and therefore I remained calm."

- **How you dealt with the situation (if appropriate):**

"I did not shout back but tried to defuse the situation by talking with and listening to her. I took her aside and asked her about her concerns. I offered other alternatives for food if she was still hungry, which she accepted. I was able to resolve the situation, help the lady with her needs and minimise disturbance."

- **Relate to your colleague's situation:**

Was there a medical reason why the patient was not orientated or aware of what they were doing? Patients with infections, for instance, can undergo a delirium that disorientates them and leaves them susceptible to doing things they otherwise wouldn't. Did the student find out why they were angry? Did they speak to the ward nursing staff about the situation? Did they escalate it to their supervisor?

10.4 (T) Your friend comes back from successfully climbing Mount Everest. On her way to the summit she saw another climber injured and close to death. Her team decided to leave the climber so they could finish. Is this excusable?

With abstract questions like the one above, it is very easy for a candidate to give a gut response and say "yes" or "no". The interviewers aren't looking for your answer specifically, but rather the thought process that you go through to arrive at your conclusion. The question is purposely abstract, as it's unlikely candidates will have prepared an answer.

Start the answer by acknowledging that the situation is complex, particularly because there is a human life involved. Then you should begin the discussion by outlining the reasons why your friend may have chosen to abandon the injured climber. These include:

- The injured climber was already close to death and an attempt at rescue may already be futile.
- Rescuing the climber will force the team to abandon their summit attempt, which is something the team would likely have been training and preparing for over the previous months, if not years.
- Attempting a rescue may pose a significant threat to the lives of the summit team. This may be because of inadequate training, or because the time associated with the rescue would result in the entire team having to tackle changing and unfavourable weather conditions.

You should then progress to balancing your statement by discussing reasons why the act was inexcusable. These include:

- We should never abandon another person to die, even if there is only a small chance that they may survive, and all attempts at rescue should be made.
- By excusing this act, it may be that future climbers will also fail to offer help, and this may lead to a slippery slope of ethical decline.

Once you have balanced both sides of the argument, try to conclude with your position and justify it with the arguments you've made. Again, in this scenario it's not uncommon for interviewers to then push the candidate a little more by challenging their stance. Stronger candidates here will be able to acknowledge the flaws in their own arguments, be able to demonstrate empathy for both arguments, yet still balance that by defending their position.

10.5 (MMI) You have said that you do ballet. Could you tell us how you would teach us to do a basic ballet step? You have 5 minutes.

This question may sound abstract; however, teaching is an important attribute for a doctor to possess. Medicine is a career that involves lifelong learning and doctors continually teach and learn from each other. Therefore, this question is assessing whether you could break down a technique that you are experienced at to a level that someone else could learn from.

Of course it may not be ballet – this question could be asked in relation to any sport, instrument or hobby that you participate in. If you have mentioned it in your personal statement, be prepared to speak about it!

The best way to approach this question is to think of the way that you learnt the technique most successfully and to break it down into manageable steps:
"Yes, I would establish your level of ballet before commencing – I would ask whether you have learnt any ballet before or if you were a complete beginner.

I would explain to you what I was going to teach at a level appropriate for you and explain why it is an important step in ballet.

I would show you the step slowly and take you to the barre so that you could balance. We would then practise the step slowly together. As you grew more confident with the step I would encourage you to practise it on your own and then speed up the move until you felt ready to practise it in the centre. Finally we could add music."

Finish the question off with a relation to medicine and why this would make you an ideal doctor:
"Teaching is an essential skill for doctors and I have demonstrated my aptitude for teaching through my participation in training more junior ballet dancers.

I often seek feedback from the learners I interact with and it has really helped me to develop as a patient and enthusiastic teacher."

10.6   (T) What particular artwork/piece would you say represents you and why?

This seems like a strange question, but it is a good chance to show your personality and interests outside of medicine and to showcase your reflective skills.

The interviewers probably want to get a sense of who you are as a person. It is a great opportunity to relay some of the key personality traits they are looking for in their medical students. Start by thinking of your strengths (reflective, analytical, team worker…) and since art is about interpretation, you can interpret the art to suit what you want to say, in most cases.

You can choose any artist/piece; it is the explanation that will make a good answer. You might want to begin with a particular piece, how it represents some part of your personality then end with how this links to medicine. You could do this in a number of ways:

You could refer to a specific art movement, what it means to you and how it relates to your personality. For example:

Surrealism – you could say how you like to look at things from different ways, like to think outside the box, which helps you to problem-solve and reflect.

Pop art – you could say that you are very animated, highlighting your warmth, ability to work well in a team, or your communication/people skills.

Realism – you could highlight that you are hardworking, have high attention to detail, reflecting the high-quality artwork from this time.

How would these qualities help you as a doctor? For example, you can easily build rapport.

Alternatively, you could concentrate on the subject; for example, if it is an animal then you could cleverly try to link this to the desirable traits they are looking for.

An example: *"I really admire the surrealist work of Magritte so I would probably have to say the piece '**False mirror**'. I find it especially interesting how the artist depicts that things may not be as they first appear. I think this represents me because I like to think outside the box and look at things from different perspectives."*

You might want to then link this to medicine:

"…Thinking outside the box is important in medicine as holistic treatment of patients is important, and at first their reason for seeing you may not be obvious."

TOP TIP   Even if you know nothing about art, you can still choose a famous picture (everyone's heard of at least one!) and think creatively about how it could represent you.

10.7 (T) What are your thoughts on the use of art in a hospital setting?

This question is asking you to discuss something fairly abstract and something you may not be entirely familiar with. You could start by mentioning what possible types of art can be used in hospitals:

- Paintings – maybe from local artists or schoolchildren
- Bright wall colours may be classed as artistic
- Sculptures e.g. in any outdoor areas or the atrium.

You can then say where art could be used or where you have seen any (if applicable):

- Children's ward e.g. cartoons on walls may help to calm children and also entertain them
- Corridors
- Waiting rooms and relatives' rooms.

Even if you are unsure of what exactly the interviewers are 'getting at' you will perform well in most questions by adopting a 'pros and cons' type of approach:

Pros:

- May improve patient and staff mood. Perhaps it may have a healing effect on ill patients?
- Can give patients/relatives something to focus on when waiting
- More aesthetically pleasing
- Gives sense of pride to artists to see their work displayed where it may help others.

Cons:

- Infection control risk – could sculptures and paintings harbour dust and spread infection?
- Costly (unless donated) – money that could be better spent on patient treatment.

Finish off by giving your opinion: do you think art should be used within a hospital? Both yes and no are valid answers, but make sure you justify your answer.

If you think art should not be used in a hospital but could be useful in other areas of healthcare e.g. general practice or drop-in centres, you could mention this.

10.8 (T) Let's assume consultant doctors were paid £30 000 per annum. Do you still want to be a doctor? What if they were paid minimum wage?

This is a challenging question. Essentially they want to know if you are doing it for the money. If not, are you prepared to put yourself through the rigour of medical school and postgraduate training for a minimum wage salary?

Start by addressing the question. For example:
"This is a difficult question because having a reasonable amount of money is required so that you don't have to worry about the basic necessities of life such as providing for your family and paying the bills, etc."

Next make it very clear you are not in it for the money. For example:
"I am not and have never been obsessed with making money. If I was, I think there are far easier options to make money than putting myself through the rigour of medical school and postgraduate training. From my work experience I realised I love the practice of clinical medicine and more importantly I will be happy to practise as a doctor and really enjoy what I do. I think this is crucial because if you don't love what you do, it will show in your performance and you will find it difficult to push yourself to your potential and go that extra mile for patients, when required."

Now go back to the original question. For example:
"Because I love the subject and truly believe I will be a competent, effective doctor, I think I would be happy with a salary of £30 000. That salary would be sufficient to sustain my lifestyle. However, at minimum wage, even though I would like to practise as a doctor, that salary would mean I would not be financially free – especially given the cost associated with studying medicine at an undergraduate and postgraduate level. This may have an effect on my personal and professional life and I don't think I would be very happy or be able to provide for my family. Therefore if a consultant salary was minimum wage, I would have to rethink my career aspirations simply because it would be a struggle financially, especially with a family."

The following points should be addressed when answering this question:
- Acknowledge that you understand a reasonable salary is important in life. This shows that you are not naïve.
- Let them know you are not in it for the money and that you want to be a doctor because you love the practice of clinical medicine.
- Don't be afraid to say you won't be a consultant doctor for minimum wage. If you ask consultants now if they would do it for minimum wage the vast majority would probably say no!

10.9 **(MMI) You are a consultant doctor and your patient requests you to stop life-saving treatment and just pray for them to get better. Please discuss this with the patient, who will be played by an actor. You have 7 minutes.**

From the outset there are two important points you should understand:

- A competent adult patient who has **mental capacity** has the right to withdraw life-saving treatment.
- A patient does not necessarily have the right to request a particular treatment. The doctor decides the treatment that is given.

You also need to know what 'mental capacity' is. It would be useful to read the Mental Capacity Act. A person is said to have full mental capacity if they can:

- Understand the information relevant to the decision
- Retain that information
- Use or weigh up that information as part of the process of making the decision
- Communicate their decision.

With regard to praying for your patient, this is a difficult question and largely depends on your personal views of what your job is as a physician and your belief in prayer. Even if you are an atheist it may be comforting for the patient if you say you will pray for them.

Remember a state of health is not just physical wellbeing but also mental and spiritual.

However, if you are not comfortable or willing to do this you are within your rights to refuse. You could suggest alternatives, such as asking the hospital chaplain to visit them or speaking to their own religious leader to arrange a hospital visit.

After you have explained the background of what capacity is and the issues surrounding treatment refusal, you need to explain to the patient in a way they fully understand what will happen if they refuse treatment, explain why you are offering them the treatment you recommend and listen to their reasons for refusal. Don't assume their reasons are not rational – listen very carefully.

You should never coerce a patient into accepting any form of treatment even if that treatment will save their life. A patient with capacity has every right to decide what happens to their body.

10.10   (T) What aspects of your life are you most proud of?

This is a less conventional question that may surprise the candidate, designed to establish interests outside medicine/education. Because of the very nature of the question, a 'perfect' answer is impossible to prepare. However, by following the format of the answer below, a well-prepared candidate could demonstrate altruistic personality traits as well as a commitment to academic study, two traits that will certainly impress the interviewers.

In order to approach this question effectively, you could split your answer into two sections:
1. Addressing an aspect of your life outside academia
2. An aspect of your educational life.

A good example would read as follows:

"I feel it is important to have a sense of pride in one's achievements, and I have two aspects of my life I would like to discuss. Firstly, I am proud of my summer job working in a nursing home – it has given me an insight into how a caring approach can really make a difference to the lives of others, and reinforced my belief that the patient should be at the centre of everything a doctor does.

Secondly, in the course of the last academic year, my classmates and I won an analytical chemistry competition, competing in a number of heats against other schools to win a monetary prize for our school. This experience allowed me to test my team working ability in a pressured environment, a skill I know will be required of me if I am to become a doctor."

Remember what characteristics the people in charge of medical school admissions are looking for: empathy, an altruistic personality, team working, the ability to learn from experiences and a real commitment to lifelong learning.

It is important to be aware of what you are applying for, and to relate your answer in some way to the medical profession. Other things you may wish to mention are volunteer work of any description (helping with a homework club, sports coaching, working in a charity shop), anything you did as part of a team (winning a cup with a sports team, a charity fundraiser with a school/youth group, a concert with a school orchestra) and achievements that highlight a commitment to academia (excellent results in exams, attendance at summer schools).

10.11 *(MMI) You are in a boat on a lake and there's a rock on the boat. If you throw the rock out of the boat, how will the level of the water change? You have 5 minutes to consider your answer (you are free to use the pen and paper provided). You will then be asked to present your answer to the interviewer.*

Many interviewees will read this question and immediately panic, especially if you have not recently studied maths or physics at school. Getting the right answer is not essential to the station, but approaching it in a systematic and logical manner is more important. It is unlikely that you will be asked this exact question but instead it is important to develop a logical approach to any 'startling' question.

A stepwise approach would be:
- **An object will float on water if it is less dense than water**, such as a piece of polystyrene or the boat. When any object floats on water, it displaces its own *mass* in the water. If our rock weighs 1kg, it will displace 1kg of water whilst in the boat.
- **An object will sink in water if it has a greater density than water**, such as an anvil or the rock. When any object sinks in water, it displaces its own *volume* in the water. If our rock has a volume of 1L, it will displace 1L of water whilst in the water.
- Therefore, **when the rock is in the boat it will displace an equivalent mass of water, yet when it sinks in the lake it will displace an equivalent volume of water.**
- **A rock on its own has a greater density than water**, so when the rock goes from the boat to the lake, less water is displaced than before. The water level will go down.

To further explain this, here is an example:
- A rock has a volume of 500ml and has a mass of 1kg (remember that 1L of water has a 1kg mass).
- When in the boat, the rock displaces an equivalent mass of water (which is 1L).
- When in the lake, the rock displaces its own volume in the water (which is 500ml).
- When the rock is thrown from boat to water, the water level will therefore go down by 500ml.

As mentioned earlier, you do not necessarily need to get the correct answer at this station to do well. Being systematic and logical with your thinking and reasoning will be much more important to show the interviewer. The interviewer may even prompt you at each stage, but it would be even better if you could answer it without prompting.

10.12   (T) *What is the most recent non-medical book you have read?*

This may seem like a random question but can help to assess a candidate's interests outside of academia and their ability to think on their feet. It is likely this may be followed up with questions such as: could you describe the basic plot of the book? What did you take/learn from the book?

It is impossible to predict the questions you could be asked about the book you have read, but some general guidance is as follows:

Firstly, make sure you are maintaining some diversity to your interests and not purely focusing on 'what will look good on a personal statement'. It is definitely worth reading some medicine-related books to gain some insight into the medical world but don't feel you can't read anything else. It may not be reading, but having an outlet for stress or an immersive activity is an invaluable tool as a medical student. Your hobbies will equip you with skills to help with your career as well as protect you from burnout.

Secondly, don't be afraid to be honest. This may mean admitting you can't remember, or that the last book you read was the reference book from GCSE English. You won't get extra marks if you say you're reading *War and Peace*, but you may make a bad impression if you can't describe a book well, either because you haven't actually read it or read it just because you thought 'it would sound good in an interview'.

When describing a book, just like any other interview question, take your time. This is a great opportunity to showcase the descriptive skills you will use every day as a doctor to present patients to colleagues or to explain information to patients. The key is to have a good structure, starting with some basic information to set the scene, such as whether it is fiction or non-fiction and where it is set. From there you can go into more detail, again trying to be systematic and clear.

10.13   (T) How many piano tuners are there in the USA?

At first, this kind of question will most likely throw you, but try not to panic!

Interviewers may choose to throw in a question similar to this and its main purpose is to test your logic and reasoning skills. The thing to remember is, you are not expected to pull a number or one-word answer out of thin air!

Start with the basics. How many people are there living in the USA? Take an approximate guess of 300 million. This doesn't have to be exactly right, just roughly in the right region.

Let's say then, on average, there are four people in a family. That means there are about 75 million families living in the USA. How many of these families might own a piano? Roughly, you could say about 10% of them own one. This means that around 7.5 million families own a piano and so there are about 7.5 million pianos that need tuning in the USA.

Now you need to think about how many piano tuners are actually required.

On average, let's assume that a piano tuner can tune 5 pianos a day and that they work 5 days a week, 50 weeks of the year. From these numbers, you can work out that one piano tuner can tune 1250 pianos over the course of one year (52 weeks). Therefore, we can calculate the following:

7.5 million/1250 = 6000

This gives you your final rough figure of around 6000 piano tuners required in the USA.

The interviewers are not necessarily interested in how close to the true value your own answer is. They want to see that you are able to logically reason your way through a completely strange scenario or challenge, as this is an important skill required of a future doctor. As long as you talk through your thinking, they will be impressed!

10.14 *(MMI) You lead a team of interviewers selecting medical school students. A new interviewer has just been recruited. Please explain to the interviewer the characteristics and qualities you would look for, and why, when interviewing potential medical school students. You will be asked to communicate with an actor who will play the new interviewer. You have 6 minutes to complete the station.*

This station is testing your knowledge on the qualities that you are trying to demonstrate yourself to the interview panels. The characteristics are wide-ranging – from your professional to personal attributes.

Although there are many attributes that you may bring up, try to ensure that essentials aren't missed – such as team player, and the ability to demonstrate empathy.

- **Introduce yourself, and give your role:**
  "Hello, I am Kirstin, and I am team leader for medical interviewers. Can I check what your name is please?"
- **Outline your plan for the conversation:**
  "I will be telling you about the characteristics we look for when interviewing medical students."
- **Ask if they have any prior experience to enable you to pitch your conversation accordingly:**
  "Have you interviewed at medical schools, or elsewhere, before?"
- **Explain that first impressions count:** *"The student should be dressed appropriately for the situation, to ensure they appreciate the seriousness of the situation. An overly casual look may reflect otherwise."*
- **Then, start bringing up attributes, as well as a short explanation of why they are important:** *"A student should be realistic about the challenges of the career as well as the positives, so that they are prepared for the coming obstacles."*
- **Another example might be:** *"The student should be able to clearly display empathy when referring to patients in difficult situations. Every doctor must have empathy, because they are often in contact with vulnerable patients in difficult situations."*
- **Go over three to four attributes that you think are the most important for a potential medical student to display.**
- **Stay clear of the common pitfall of providing a list of attributes with no explanation.**
- **Conclude professionally:** *"Now that I have gone through some characteristics that we look for in a medical student, do you have any questions?"*
- **Thank the new interviewer:** *"Thank you for coming today and we look forward to working with you."*

10.15 (MMI) Which has been the greatest medical advance – antibiotics, chemotherapy or X-rays? You will have 5 minutes to present your answer to the interviewer.

This question is designed to assess your reasoning skills, rather than your knowledge. The interviewer expects you to present both sides of an argument and derive a logical conclusion.

> **TOP TIP** The natural approach by applicants is to reel off all their knowledge about each topic in a panic. Take 30 seconds to think of two or three bullet points on each topic and develop your arguments. When making a comparison, try to use a specific measure e.g. number of lives saved or improvement in quality of life, to provide quantitative evidence behind each argument.

Antibiotics:
- The widespread use of antibiotics since the 1940s has saved countless lives.
- At the start of the 20th century, infectious diseases were responsible for the majority of deaths in the world; currently, non-communicable diseases such as heart disease, stroke and chronic lung disease have surpassed infectious diseases as the leading causes of death.
- It is difficult to determine the precise impact of antibiotics, as the decline in the prevalence of infectious disease is also affected by improved hygiene and vaccinations.
- The widespread development of antibiotic resistance causes concern about the usefulness of antibiotics in the future.

Chemotherapy:
- Since the development of chemotherapy, previously fatal conditions such as childhood acute lymphoblastic leukaemia, Hodgkin's lymphoma and testicular cancer are now curable.
- Chemotherapy can also improve survival chances following surgery for high-risk cancers e.g. breast.
- The overall impact of chemotherapy on cancer survival is difficult to gauge as other determinants such as screening, prevention (e.g. anti-smoking campaigns) and detection have also had an effect.

X-rays:
- The discovery of X-rays in 1895 led to the growth of the medical imaging field.
- X-rays have paved the way for computed tomography (CT), fluoroscopy, mammography and angiography imaging modalities.
- The harmful effects of X-ray radiation exposure have even been harnessed to produce targeted radiotherapy treatments.

10.16 **(T) You are offered a fully paid scholarship to study medicine. However, the company giving you this scholarship is an unethical commercial company whose products have destroyed thousands of lives. Without this scholarship, you would not be able to afford to study medicine. Would you take the scholarship?**

Studying medicine is a dream come true for many students. Some might be fortunate to come from very financially secure backgrounds. For others, the course fees, living costs and mandatory books/equipment costs may make studying medicine a difficult choice. This scenario is fictional but raises some important ethical challenges. You must evaluate the pros and cons of seeking a scholarship from the unscrupulous company and make a decision about whether you would accept it.

Pros:
- If you don't accept the money from the company it may be spent on a much less worthy cause, or a cause that could even adversely affect humanity.
- By accepting the grant it may give you the option to discuss with or report back to company officials. It may therefore be an opportunity to reason with them about their poor humanitarian record.
- It will allow you to study medicine without distraction and as such get much more out of your course. This may allow you to be a better doctor.

Cons:
- The goal of the company is likely to be to deliver a profit to its shareholders. You may feel coerced into acting unethically (but in the company's favour) at some point in the future because of your financial links.
- Regardless of whether you ever act unethically or not, patients may find it difficult to trust a doctor if they find out they have financial links to an unethical company. This may harm the doctor–patient relationship.

A balanced answer in this scenario might be to highlight the pros and cons above. You could then explain you would decline the financial support from the company and highlight the other avenues for financial support that exist (student loans, professional loans, ordinary bank loans, part-time jobs, bursaries from universities...).

The interviewer may raise an issue with part-time jobs and the negative impact they may have on your ability to commit time to studying. You can stress how much effort you would put into your studies and that they would definitely come first. You can point out that some students successfully balance a part-time job and medicine. You can even highlight, with an example, how you have managed your time very well in the past.

Chapter 11 | Knowledge of the course

11.1 (T) Why do you want to study at this medical school?

This is a common question frequently asked in both styles of interview. It is a relatively straightforward question that allows candidates to settle into the interview process. During your interview preparation, it may be useful to organise your reasons into broader categories for simplicity, e.g.:

- Course (curriculum, PBL, lecture-based, early clinical experience, workshops, small group tutorials)
- Medical school (location, distance from hospital site, facilities)
- University (campus, leisure facilities, clubs and societies)
- City (current home, living and travel arrangements, leisure activities).

You can select one or two examples from each category for a broad list of reasons. For example, you may choose the following from the first category:

"I have attended an open day at this medical school, and the emphasis of the course on gaining early clinical experience appealed greatly to me as I know from past experience that I learn most effectively through experience."

This answer demonstrates your motivation for applying to this medical school, whilst supporting your answer with evidence of a genuine effort to research your choice, e.g. attending an open day. Moreover, it also shows the interview panel that you have personal insight into your preferred learning style, and such self-awareness is a useful quality to possess in medicine.

Other examples may include:

"I was impressed with the anatomy workshops during the open day, because they provide a visual and hands-on approach to learning difficult concepts, which, from my previous experiences, helps expand on didactic teaching."

"I spent a week exploring the city earlier this year, and I have found that, due to the medical school's central location in the city, it is conveniently situated within a short distance of two large teaching hospitals and several local GP practices, which I find very convenient."

Note that these examples all link your choice to personal reasons, which helps to create a genuine answer and also demonstrates that a certain level of thought and research has gone into your decision.

TOP TIP Be aware that the interview panel may very well put you on the spot depending on the reason that you give, e.g. *"Why not other medical schools that offer a PBL course?"* To avoid this potentially awkward situation, be prepared to give several different reasons and explain that it is the combination of factors that collectively influenced your final decision.

11.2   (T) What attracts you the most and the least about this medical school?

In this question you need to be tactful. Try to use the positive points to supersede any negative points. Start by stating the positive points. Here are some ideas:

- The style of the course suits you. Justify how it suits you: is the course problem-based or traditional? Does it have a lot of practical sessions or does it have an allocated time period to do research?
- The medical school and teaching hospitals have a good reputation. Explain where you have heard this from: was it from current students, other doctors or ranking tables?
- You liked the feel you got when you visited the school. Points such as: people were friendly, great facilities, approachable staff.
- You have family or friends close by and like the area. For example: you like living in a big city, access to the airport, good transport links to university and hospitals.
- The medical school has a wide variety of activities to get involved in that you would really enjoy, for example strong sports teams, choir, debating, charity work, climbing and drama.

After giving the interviewer the positive points that attracted you to their university you can begin to address what you don't like about it.

TOP TIP Try to avoid saying that there is nothing negative about the medical school, as it doesn't sound like you're being honest and may come across as though you haven't put much thought into it.

One approach is to talk about things that aren't really faults of the medical school, such as that the university is far away from your family. Here is another approach, which avoids insulting the medical school whilst still addressing that fact that you have thought about the negatives:

"I have done a lot of research into various medical schools and found this medical school to be the most suited to me. I am sure that during my studies I will come across some negative aspects; however, so far there is nothing that has really discouraged me. It seems like an excellent medical school and all the students I have spoken to have very positive feedback so I am really looking forward to joining."

It is a good idea to discuss the positive points first and then only briefly mention the negatives. You can then close it by focusing on positive points again. This will show the interviewer that you have put some thought into picking this particular medical school and that you are passionate about studying there.

11.3 (T) What do you not like about this course?

Unlike previous questions this question exclusively asks which aspects of the course you see as a negative. Like other questions, however, it is still seeking to establish how much you know about the course, and assessing whether you acknowledge that there may be components of the degree that you would rather not do or will find challenging. Again, like previous questions, a terrible way to answer this question is to say, *"There is nothing I wouldn't like about this course."* This type of answer doesn't demonstrate insight. Nor does it demonstrate that you have an understanding of the course.

It is a good idea to read the literature available on each course thoroughly before the day of your interview. This may be found on the medical school website. It is even more impressive if you can say that you have discussed the medical school with current medical students and recent graduates to determine what the course is 'really like'.

You may find aspects of the course (like the examples below) that you do not like the sound of:

- *"The course involves using cadaveric material as an anatomy teaching aid. I have never seen a dead body before, so I am nervous as to how I may react. However, I understand that our exposure will progress slowly and I will ensure my anatomy knowledge is exemplary, to allow me to look at the material as a teaching aid and focus on the learning gained from the activity."*
- *"From the information I have read, I understand that for our clinical placements, we could be two hours away from the university and in a more remote area. I would rather not be placed this far away; however, if I took every opportunity to see the more rare diseases while I was at the university hospital I could use the rural placement to consolidate my knowledge on the more common diseases. I would also use the opportunity to observe how healthcare differs in its delivery between more remote and urban areas."*

You should put a positive slant on the question to demonstrate that despite things you wouldn't like, it remains the course for you:

"Despite there being some aspects that I would find challenging, I would relish the opportunity to study here, especially given the freedom in pursuing cardiovascular physiology in the student-selected components and the more traditional approach to the teaching of basic sciences, which fits with my learning style."

11.4 (T) What qualities do you possess that would make you well suited for the problem-based learning (PBL) environment?

> **TOP TIP** PBL was developed at McMaster University Medical School in Canada in the 1960s and has become a popular teaching method adopted by many medical schools in the UK. Students work in small groups (usually around ten students) with a tutor to read through a new clinical case each week. The students collectively form a list of questions or learning points to research throughout the week. The group meet again almost a week later to discuss what they have learnt, with the tutor present to clarify information. Some medical schools provide supporting lectures and practical sessions, whereas others do not.

This question offers the chance to demonstrate your knowledge of the PBL style of teaching. Moreover, it offers you the opportunity to specifically state why you would be ideal as a medical student on a PBL course.

PBL courses are better suited to some than others, and you will likely have asked yourself if this course style is suitable for you. If you haven't, start thinking about questions such as:
- Do you enjoy working in groups?
- Does it make learning more memorable for you?
- What have you gained from working in a group setting in the past, and what roles did you play?

These are all questions that you may need to think about before formulating your answer to this question.

As with any group situation, it is important to be both an active listener and contributor. Some PBL groups will appoint a 'chair' who facilitates or drives the discussion, and a scribe who makes the session interactive by using audio-visual systems, 'smartboards', etc. You will likely serve one or both of these roles during your time as a PBL member. Try not to be too specific towards either of these roles in your answer, as it is better to answer it as a general PBL member. All PBL members, first and foremost, must be engaged and come prepared to the session. It is very obvious when an individual isn't able to follow a discussion due to not completing the learning objectives.

Contributing fairly to the discussion, asking questions to further the discussion (particularly to quieter members of the group) and being respectful to your PBL members are all key requirements for an effective working group. To this end, you must possess some basic characteristics that would make anyone suitable for PBL – bring driven/self-motivated, encouraging and supportive of your peers, patient and understanding of the group dynamic. Everyone has something unique that they bring to the group, whether it is a penchant for keeping the group organised or someone who finds new resources to meet learning objectives. Think about any of your personal strengths, how you can apply them to PBL, and it will give your answer a unique twist.

11.5   (T) What are the disadvantages of problem-based learning (PBL)?

The aim of this question is to see what you know about PBL and if you understand what it involves. If you get a question like this, it will likely be from a medical school offering a PBL medical course. Your answer to this question may need to be tailored depending on the medical school you are being interviewed by. You need to make sure you aren't too negative about the course you are applying to but that doesn't mean that you shouldn't mention a certain aspect of the course that you think might be a negative.

You can start by stating your opinion on PBL overall (this should be a positive opinion if you are applying for a PBL course).

You need to show that you know what is involved, perhaps: *"I have spent a long time weighing up the positives and negatives of both traditional and problem-based learning courses and I have come to the conclusion that problem-based learning is more suited to my personality and style of learning..."*

You can list some potential disadvantages of a PBL course. If you think something may be considered negative, but you think it is actually a positive, say why – but don't be cheesy! You can also mention ways in which these 'negatives' are tackled – this shows deeper understanding of PBL:

- *Students can have difficulties knowing how much detail they need to know.*
  - Groups are guided by facilitators – different medical schools do this differently so it is important to mention how they guide students in this regard.
- *Students can find it difficult to understand 'what' they need to know.*
  - Most PBL medical schools provide students with a list of learning outcomes and have tutors/facilitators whom students ask for guidance/help.
- *Students are responsible for their own learning.*
  - Information is not spoon-fed. Students must do the work themselves. If this is not done consistently then it is easy to fall behind.
- *There is some evidence that less knowledge is gained.*
  - However, some evidence shows that more of the information is retained.
- PBL is very different from school and may be difficult to adapt to.
- PBL can be time-consuming as you need to go away and find all of the information for yourself and then learn it.
  - If you can manage time effectively this shouldn't be a problem.
- PBL is costly to administer as a medical school due to small group work, requiring more staff as facilitators and more rooms.

It is important to finish on a high note: perhaps mention some of the positives and make sure you finish by saying that PBL is still right for you, if you are applying to a PBL medical school!

11.6 (T) This course relies heavily on self-directed learning (SDL). Can you give us an example of a time where you had to complete a task with minimal supervision or prior knowledge?

Some PBL courses require a high degree of 'self-directed' learning and you are expected to meet your own learning objectives through self-study. This differs vastly from many students' A level experience.

Think about a situation in which you had to complete a task, but were given minimal instruction. Alternatively, you can select a situation that you were entirely new to, and show how you coped to complete the specified task. The situation you choose should explain the following components:

- How you were assigned the task, and what previous knowledge you had
- What your responsibilities were, and if you had ever done anything similar
- How you approached the task and planned to carry it out
- What the outcome was, and your reflections on what worked well, and what didn't.

See the following scenario as an example (using the '**BARL**' technique):

Background: I was an A level student and had just been selected as the assistant stage manager for a production at the local community theatre. Although I had no previous experience in managing a play, I was enthusiastic about the new experience. On my first day, I was a little overwhelmed with the vast amount of information that I was given and I found one task quite daunting – coming up with a programme for the entire show.

Action: Having never done this before, I expressed this to the director who gave a quick overview of what she would like to be included, and sent me off to sort the rest myself. I decided to plan out how to approach the programme design. First, I searched for guidance online on what theatre programmes contain, and made a list of headings and information I would like to provide on the pamphlet. Next, I downloaded programme templates and designed a few mock-ups (which I found particularly fun!). I met with the casting and screenplay leads to finalise the show dates and the list of cast members.

Result: I drafted a programme and presented it to the director, who was impressed with my work. After some minor adjustments my finalised programme was submitted for printing. The performances even received coverage in a national magazine.

Link to medicine: I learnt about the importance of working with others to produce a successful programme. Having finished this task as an assistant manager, I feel more prepared and able to take on new experiences as a medical student.

11.7 (T) What are the advantages of PBL after graduation and how does PBL learning equip you for being a doctor?

It is important that you know which method of teaching the school that you are attending for interview uses. This question is different to other PBL questions in that it is specifically asking how it will help **after** graduation.

Advantages of PBL in equipping you for postgraduate medical practice:
- Promotes self-motivation to learn independently – this is key as a doctor because postgraduate exams (such as those set by the Royal Colleges and required to progress in a specialty) are often not accompanied by specific lectures and require the doctor to learn the material themselves
- Encourages self-directed learning
- Teaches students to identify appropriate learning resources – especially useful when you are a doctor since you will be expected to learn about new conditions without the luxury of being 'spoon-fed' in the medium of lectures
- Encourages learning from experience which is a daily occurrence as a doctor
- Integrates knowledge with practice: purported to help doctors recall relevant information when they are in a real-life scenario that requires that knowledge
- Equips doctors with problem analysing and solving skills to deal with real-life situations
- Develops teamwork and communication skills – essential in the workplace as a doctor.

A good example answer would be:
"There are many advantages to studying on a PBL course over one using traditional teaching methods. PBL allows students to decide what is important for them to learn in certain scenarios, which then motivates the student to study. The student will need to identify appropriate learning resources to complete their studying. Identifying learning needs and knowing where to find high-quality information is vital when you are a doctor. This is because medical practice changes rapidly and doctors are required to keep their skills and knowledge up to date without regular lectures or tutorials. In addition, when working for postgraduate exams there is often little direct teaching and doctors have to be able to seek appropriate resources from which to learn."

11.8   (T) What do you think are the negatives of studying in east London?

Although this may seem like a relatively straightforward question about the university, and its location, it is important to think to yourself about what is actually required of you.

If you are asked such a question, the interviewer is probably already aware of the negatives.

This question could be adapted to any region or city in the country. You need to be aware about all aspects of the course and medical school, especially if it is in an area that may not be particularly glamorous. Medical schools come in all forms. Perhaps your chosen medical school is located in the countryside with a relatively small population or it could be in inner city London.

Think about what kind of things are different in inner cities compared to other places.

Inner city populations tend to be more multicultural and you may even face language differences.

If your medical school is located in the countryside close to a relatively small town then you may not see as many different conditions and infections as you would in the city. However, you may see a different spectrum of disease e.g. lung conditions caused by the dust involved in farming.

It is important to look at both the negative and positive aspects of your medical school and be prepared to answer anything about the course or university.

"East London has a large population of people from different cultures. As a medical student I may come across people who are unable to speak English and therefore communication would be difficult. Although in an ideal situation I would have an interpreter available, I understand that this is not always the case. Another challenge I could potentially face is dealing with people who have specific health beliefs that may not complement modern medicine."

Now talk about how some of these may actually be positives.

You have previously talked about cultural and language barriers, but these are great learning points and may enrich your experience. You will become familiar with treating patients who do not believe in the same things as you.

You can also mention some of the extra-curricular benefits of living in certain areas.

11.9 (T) What do you see as the benefits of studying medicine in south-east London?

Similar to the previous question, this one applies to just a few universities. However, the structure of the answer below can be applied to all similar questions, for those aiming for to study in south-west England, the north-east or anywhere in between.

You should have some basic knowledge of what could be called the 'medical geography' of the area. Which hospitals are nearby? Which are the teaching hospitals and which are less well-known District General Hospitals (DGHs)? Is primary care generally delivered by individual GP surgeries, or are there large polyclinics to serve the population? It is vital to demonstrate an understanding of the area beyond just medical facilities. Is the area affluent, deprived or mixed? Is the population ethnically diverse or uniform? How may this affect the burden of disease in the area and the cases you may see on placements?

In answering this question about south-east London I would recognise that three excellent teaching hospitals are within very close proximity, and that perhaps the UK's foremost psychiatric institute is closely linked to one of the medical schools in the area. As discussed in the previous question, south-east London is extremely diverse, with many deprived neighbourhoods in close proximity to extremely affluent postcodes. A vast number of different ethnic minorities have made this part of London home, whilst there are also large numbers of wealthier commuters of all backgrounds in the borough. This spectrum of society brings many challenges to healthcare, but also many educational benefits to the medical student. Conditions not normally seen in Britain may be prevalent in those moving to the region from other international locations. At the same time exposure to the consumer demands of the commuter population (the 'worried well') may be equally educational, teaching students to hone their negotiating skills, rather than using a more didactic 'traditional doctor–patient' approach. It may be that on general practice placement a medical student in one of these areas observes doctors carefully not prescribing antibiotics and not referring patients to specialists, perhaps finding that reassurance is a better use of resources than expensive medicines, tests and further appointments.

It would be remiss to not make a point of the other countless opportunities a city like London affords you to develop into a well-rounded doctor. Your interview is your chance to show that you are a balanced individual – your academic track record should speak for itself. It is essential that you show that there is so much more to life than locking oneself away in the library and studying all the time. Whatever your extra-curricular passion there is some way to pursue it. The extra educational opportunities hosted by various medical and scientific institutions should also be mentioned – the Royal Society of Medicine, the Wellcome Collection, all of the Royal Colleges. Almost all have some sort of student membership grade or other ways of getting involved with their programmes of events.

11.10 (T) Some medical schools introduce clinical medicine very early in the course. Why do you think this medical school doesn't?

Clearly there are many different ways of structuring medical degree courses, each with their own benefits and downsides. The main reason a university would choose a programme that focuses almost entirely on theory in the earlier years of the course is that the faculty feel it may better prepare students for clinical studies, having had sound academic foundations already well established. The question should be taken not as an opportunity to debate educational theory and policy, rather it should be taken as an ideal time to show that you can see both sides of an argument, and are well aware of the approach that this particular institution has taken. This demonstrates that you have a serious interest in the institution and have enough initiative to research a topic of (considerable) interest to yourself.

If you are particularly enthusiastic about gaining some experience of interacting with patients in a clinical setting, this question should lead you to mention some of the work experience you have already undertaken, and you could demonstrate your initiative by letting the interview panel know about some of the extra-curricular activities you have planned. Part-time first aid work is a very popular means that some medical students use to help pay the rent and also give some relevance and context to the many hours of somewhat dry lectures that must be endured.

TOP TIP You don't have to have an entirely unique answer to every question in this book, since you're unlikely to be asked all of them. You can also answer this question with some of the points that have been raised in previous questions about self-directed learning and problem-based learning. What is important is that you can speak eloquently and intellectually about each topic. By having a well-structured response in mind you can answer many of these questions, which are quite similar. However, if you are asked two similar questions in your interview, it is important to answer each in a unique way.

11.11 (T) From what you understand, what do you think will be the biggest challenge for you while studying medicine?

This question is looking to assess your awareness about what medicine involves. Listen to the question carefully – it is different to questions that ask about the challenges of a career as a doctor. As such, you should tailor your answer appropriately. You should show that you have looked at what studying medicine is like and are aware of any difficulties you might face at the medical school you are applying for.

You could start off this question by demonstrating that you have done some research into what medicine is like. Some examples are: talking to medical students, attending a summer school, online resources, books or talking to doctors on your work experience. This will show you have a keen interest in medicine and that after having looked into the course, you still want to pursue it.

You should then give a feature of the course that you may find challenging. The answer will be personal to you, but below you will find examples of the difficulties faced by medical students. You should then say how you think you will find a solution to the challenges you will face:

- **The quantity of work can be overwhelming**
  - Improve and work on time management skills. Keep on top of work throughout the year.
- **Treating very sick patients can be challenging to deal with emotionally**
  - Talk to other medical students or staff members about how best to manage this. Give an example of a coping mechanism that works for you.
- **It can be stressful**
  - What do you do to relieve stress? This may be exercise, watching your favourite TV programme or another hobby e.g. painting.
- **Requires independent learning**
  - You could mention a situation where you have had to work independently and apply this to your medical career e.g. a project at sixth form, revision for exams, etc.
- **Moving away from home for the first time**
  - Give an example of a time when you have been away from home and mention how you found this, and how you coped. If you have never been away from home, say this, and suggest a way in which you will deal with this e.g. plan visits home, calling home regularly.

Finish by saying that you have understood what is required of a medical student and that you are aware of the difficulties. Make sure the interviewer knows that even with these challenges, medicine is still what you want to do!

11.12 *(MMI) You are a first-year medical student and a prospective student from your home town asks you for advice on the course. They are unsure what exactly an intercalated BSc entails. Please discuss with the prospective student (who will be played by an actor) your thoughts on undertaking an intercalated BSc. You have 7 minutes to complete this station.*

For every medical school interview you attend, regardless of whether it involves traditional or multiple mini interviews, it is important to know the structure of the medical school curriculum. Medical education is constantly evolving and you should know how the medical school you are applying to has structured their course.

Intercalated BSc programmes form a large part of many medical school curricula. Even if you do not know whether you want to undertake one at the stage of your interview, make sure you know about the scheme. Information on the intercalated BSc programmes can be found easily for most medical schools, via their prospectus, website, or even ringing up their offices.

There are pros and cons to undertaking an intercalated year and it will be important to convey both these sides in your answer at this station:
Pros:
- Allows a student to explore a subject outside of the normal curriculum in a topic of medicine they find interesting
- They offer a chance to explore future possible career options
- Having an additional degree, which can be completed in one year, can give your CV a competitive edge
- There are currently additional points available for those with an additional degree when applying for foundation year jobs, as well as in further training
- Students may have an opportunity to explore new activities or hobbies, which otherwise they may not have been able to do on the medical course

Cons:
- Taking another year in education comes with financial implications
- It adds an additional year to your medical training, so your training overall will take longer.
- Some individuals simply do not enjoy research and research projects, thus may find the year not enjoyable or beneficial.

11.13 (T) This course involves a lot of contact hours at university and on placement. Do you think you'll have time to keep up any hobbies/interests?

First and foremost, the answer to this question should be "Yes!"

Hobbies and interests are an essential element of a good work–life balance. As a potential future doctor, you will no doubt be inundated with tasks at work and if you don't find a way to unwind, the workload could have a negative effect on your wellbeing.

In your answer, you can talk about any hobbies you might already be pursuing. This can be anything from music to sport to writing your own novel! Whether this involves being part of a team or just relaxing on your own, you should stress the importance of hobbies and interests when answering – they can help you remain healthy and happy as you follow a career that may be testing at times.

"Medicine is a rewarding yet demanding career, and the high workload could sometimes lead to a build-up of stress. To try and combat this, I feel that it is important for me to keep up with my hobbies, as it will give me a chance to relax and loosen up, especially after long, hard days at work. I have been part of a five-a-side football team for a few years now and I hope to continue playing football when I come to university, as it is something I look forward to every week."

You should also try to show some understanding of the complexity of the course – the phrasing of the question has drawn attention to this already so it is important to acknowledge how challenging it may become at times. However, the interviewers want to know that you will still try to keep up your hobbies for all the above reasons. This is the perfect opportunity to showcase your excellent time management skills!

For example:
"I understand that the course involves a lot of contact hours and that it might be difficult, at times, to keep up any extra-curricular interests that I have. However, in the past, I think that I have already shown that I can balance studies and hobbies well. I have played in a rock band for the past three years – this involved a practice at least once a week, if not more. However, these regular meetings did not affect my educational performance and I was able to achieve three As at A level while also being able to relax regularly."

11.14 (T) What is the structure of the medical course at this University? We use an 'academy-based' structure – can you describe what that means?

This question will vary depending on the university you are applying to. Ensure that you look at the curriculum before interview. The 'academy' structure is unique to some universities.

An example answer to this question may be: *"During the clinical years (Years 3–5) of the Medicine course at the University of St Wilson's, students will be provided with their clinical teaching within academies across the region.*

Students should expect to be placed in the main city of St Wilson's for half of the year and outside of St Wilson's for the other half. The other towns that students could be placed include Summershire, Wintershire, Glenautumn and Springtown. An outline of what to expect in each year includes:"

	Year	Modules	Clinical experience
Preclinical	1	Human Basis of Medicine Molecular and Cellular Basis of Medicine Systems of a Body part 1	Mainly university based. Students will observe GP consultations with patients once a week for a term.
	2	Systems of a Body parts 2 & 3 Student Selected Component (SSC) Clinical integration module	Mainly university based. The clinical integration module gives students 2–3 weeks' experience in a hospital before starting the clinical years.
Clinical	3	Medicine & Surgery part 1 Musculoskeletal Diseases, Emergency Medicine & Ophthalmology Pathology & Ethics	All year within clinical academies
	4	Obstetrics & Gynaecology and Sexual Health Psychiatry & Anaesthetics Community Health Care	All year within clinical academies
	5	Medicine & Surgery part 2 Foundation shadowing Student Selected Component	All year within clinical academies

The benefits of an academy-based structure:
- Students will experience a variety of different hospital environments, from large teaching hospitals to district general hospitals.
- Students will be required to move to and study in different cities across the region; this will mimic the movements that junior doctors will have to make in Foundation years.
- Teaching styles/facilities vary between academies, giving students a rounded experience.

11.15 **(MMI) Discuss one of your hobbies with the interviewer, and show how the skills you acquired from this activity will help you during your time as a medical student. You will be asked to communicate with an actor in this station. You have 7 minutes to complete the station.**

This is a relatively simple scenario – provided it is answered correctly. It provides the opportunity to speak about something you really care about, so choose wisely.

This question has two parts. The first concerns a hobby of your choice. This will reflect your all-round personality and abilities beyond the classroom.

The second part of the question concerns your ability to think critically to find a way to transfer skills. A model answer would be:

- Introduce yourself and your hobby: *"Hello, my name is Gemma. The hobby I will be discussing is gymnastics."*
- Explain when you started your hobby, and successes you have had in its field, if applicable: *"I started gymnastics at the age of 12, and I have been consistently training since then. I have participated in several competitions, and recently won 2nd place at the National Gymnastics Competition, in the artistic gymnastics category."*
- Now introduce attributes you believe are essential to being a successful medical student: *"As a medical student, one must be consistent, determined, and proactive."*
- Tie the two together now, by stating an attribute you have learned from your hobby, and how it will be useful as a medical student. An example might be: *"I have demonstrated my determination and proactive nature by consistently training twice a week to maintain my gymnastics level. In medicine, I recognise the importance of consistently working throughout the year to stay on top of my workload."*
- Finally, describe your hobby as an outlet to your normal daily life. Breaks from schoolwork are imperative, and it is important you recognise this, as a well-rounded individual.

11.16 (T) This medical school and the hospitals used for teaching are in an area where the majority of the residents are from certain ethnic or socioeconomic groups. What kind of healthcare issues do you think might come up often?

The important part of answering this question is to know the medical school you are applying to well! Make sure you look into where it is, who lives around it and what different ethnic or socioeconomic groups may be in that area.

Although many medical schools tend to be in large cities, there are a few that are in more rural areas, so there are obvious social and health differences in these two areas. Urban populations tend to struggle with increased psychological stress or chronic conditions such as asthma. In contrast, these are less common in rural populations, but the people living here might struggle to actually access healthcare as easily – this is known as a health inequality.

Looking at specific ethnic groups, you are probably aware of different recurring diseases all over the world. For example:
- In the UK, heart disease is one of the most common chronic conditions and causes of death.
- In China, there is a very high rate of lung cancer due to their high smoking rates.
- In Japan, the rate of gastric cancers is four times higher than the UK, potentially due to the high-salt diet.
- Individuals of South Asian descent (Pakistani, Indian, Bangladeshi, etc.) are very likely to suffer from diabetes at some point in their lives.

Certain ethnic groups may form a large part of a population and so their common health problems will come up often when you are on placement in the hospitals around them. For instance, if you were applying to a university/hospital in east London, where many individuals of South Asian descent choose to live, you would probably come across many cases of diabetes, heart disease and similar chronic conditions.

Areas that are socially or economically lacking in various ways (e.g. poorer education, lower income, higher unemployment rates, etc.) may have health issues of their own, such as:
- More unwanted pregnancies
- Higher rates of drug or alcohol abuse
- Poorer awareness of good health behaviours e.g. diet, exercise.

A lot of the time, these categories will mix – you might, for example, be applying to a university/hospital in a deprived area, where many South Asians tend to live. In this case, there will be twice as many health issues to talk about, so try to talk about as many as you can. This shows the interviewers that you're aware of all the different social categories in the area and how it could affect your work as a medical student.

11.17 (T) Do you feel cadaveric dissection is a vital component in medical education?

Your answer to this question should, of course, be personal. However, not every medical school in the country still practises dissection. You should be aware what the medical school you are interviewing at practises, and tailor your answer appropriately.

It is extremely important that medical students have a firm grasp of anatomy. How this is acquired is up for debate, and you have to decide how you learn best.

It would help to discuss the pros and cons of dissection:

Pros:

- It is an established technique of teaching, which has been used successfully for many years.
- Dissection has helped to drive research. It has resulted in increased understanding of unusual anatomical variations, and development of innovative surgical techniques.
- It is an interactive and practical way of seeing different parts of the body. Anatomy is not 2D. Seeing and interacting with it in 3D may assist in learning.
- It teaches a student basic practical skills which they may require if they want to be a surgeon.

Cons:

- Dissection has to take place in an approved building, making it very inflexible. Alternatives exist that may be more convenient, such as 3D computer programmes and plastic models.
- Some students find it difficult to learn in the environment of dissection for a multitude of reasons – the smell, the concept or the emotion of what they are doing may distract from their learning.
- Dissection is a skill and it may be argued that first-year medical students may not yet have the required skills to meaningfully and accurately dissect a cadaver. This may be further compounded by the fact that 'prosections' are often of excellent quality and can now be preserved using novel techniques. (Prosections are cadaveric specimens that have been pre-dissected by an expert to show the pertinent anatomy.)
- Donation of adequate numbers of cadavers for teaching has posed a challenge in recent years.

When you have considered both sides it is acceptable to choose either in favour of or against dissection, so long as you can justify your decision.

Chapter 12 | Medical knowledge

12.1 *(T) Clinical practice is becoming increasingly evidence-based. What are the limitations of evidence-based practice?*

This is a challenging question. It is a good idea to start with an opening statement to demonstrate that you understand the underlying principles of evidence-based practice in medicine, e.g. *"Evidence-based practice has become a fundamental part of modern medicine because it allows healthcare professionals to make clinical decisions based on reliable research."*

Now move on to the actual question itself, e.g. *"Notwithstanding this, I think there are some potential limitations to evidence-based practice. Namely, an evidence base is only ever as reliable as the clinical studies from which evidence is gathered. This itself is affected by a variety of factors, which include experimental design, population selection, sampling methods, transparency of all methods used in clinical studies, sharing of and access to results from all clinical studies without withholding of any results (which may be deemed research misconduct), etc."*

"Any evidence base is limited to the scope of our current understanding and research within the medical and scientific community, which in turn is limited by the availability and capabilities of existing research methods. However, as these are constantly evolving, our current understanding and the body of evidence gained from research are also likely to change periodically."

You should demonstrate to the interview panel that you have the ability to apply critical thinking in everyday practice. The importance of critical thinking cannot be overstated in medicine as it is an essential skill which helps guide your clinical judgment on a daily basis. Moreover, you will be required to make critical appraisals both as a medical student and doctor, which can involve appraising anything from healthcare policies to your fellow peers.

Other limitations of evidence-based practice:
- Clinical trials require patient participation, which carries potential risks such as adverse events, e.g. Northwick Park drug trial disaster in 2006.
- Possible conflicts of interest, e.g. some researchers might having financial ties to their research and its results.

As long as your suggestions are sensible and you can explain your reasoning in a logical manner, with examples, where possible, to support your answer, this should more than suffice to perform well in this question.

12.2 (T) What do you think is the most important medical discovery in the last 100–200 years?

This is an opportunity to illustrate your interest in medicine and demonstrate your knowledge in a particular area. There is not a single right answer here and you can give almost any answer as long as you can justify it appropriately. Some examples include:

- Antibiotics – the discovery of penicillin in 1928 by Alexander Fleming ultimately prevented the deaths of hundreds of men and women during World War II. After the war antibiotics became commercially available and have prevented the deaths of millions of people worldwide.
- The contraceptive pill – the commercial availability of the contraceptive pill in the late 1950s provided men and women with the ability to plan families. This has meant that women can now choose if and when they would like to start a family, making it easier for them to plan careers and for the future. Additionally, the pill has resolved many menstrual problems that previously were untreatable.
- The structure of DNA – the structure of DNA was discovered by Watson and Crick in 1953, and has since led to rapid, life-altering discoveries in genetic medicine, such as the identification of specific genes causing specific diseases. It is likely that the future of medicine will be personalised medicine and this is underpinned by the discovery by Watson and Crick.

You can then relate this back to your desire to study medicine such as:
"I have been inspired by the great discoveries made in medicine and would relish being able to participate in research, both as an undergraduate and postgraduate."

12.3   (T) When you think about yourself working as a doctor, who do you think will be the most important people in the team you will be working with?

In order to treat a patient, a whole team of people must work together in order to get the best possible result for the patient. At each stage of treatment different people will play prominent roles. Therefore, this question is assessing whether you know which people you may be working with and the importance of each of their jobs. You must emphasise that the care of patients is a team effort and highlight that you would be working alongside each of the following people:

- Medical doctors – *diagnose and treat the physical cause of illness and explain the illness progression and management to the patient and family.*
- Nurses – *observe and monitor a patient's progression, perform procedures on the ward and manage the patient's medication.*
- Physiotherapists – *help patients to physically rehabilitate after illness.*
- Occupational therapists – *provide equipment and strategies to patients to help them recover and manage independently.*
- Dieticians – *provide support and information to patients to allow them to manage their diet and nutrition.*
- Radiographers – *responsible for the investigation of a patient's illness by carrying out radiographic procedures such as X-rays, CT scans and MRI scans.*
- Speech and language therapist – *provide treatment strategies to aid with patients' communication and can perform assessments such as 'safe swallow' assessments after patients have had a stroke.*
- Porter – *responsible for the transport of patients around the hospital building for tests, procedures or relocation of wards.*
- Paramedic – *frequently first on the scene, often in an ambulance, to perform urgent investigations such as ECG and 'observations' such as heart rate and blood pressure. They are responsible for rapid escalation of care to another centre such as the local hospital or a specialist centre.*

12.4   (T) What is the biological mechanism of a heart attack?

This would be a harsh question, but if you get a question like this and you don't know the answer then you should say so and then explain what you do know and attempt to use your deductive reasoning to make educated statements.

> **TOP TIP**   Remember – you're applying for medical school (you're not a cardiologist yet!).
> The interviewer won't be expecting a PhD level answer – just one that demonstrates that you have a genuine interest in medicine.

You should start by saying what a heart attack is. For example, you could say *"A heart attack is not actually a medical term so it could apply to lots of things. However, it is usually describing a 'myocardial infarction'; this is when the blood flow to the heart muscle is reduced, usually due to a blocked coronary artery."*

You can then go on to explain in stages the processes that are involved:
- There is a narrowing of the coronary arteries.
- This is caused by the build-up of fatty plaques in their walls.
- Due to the narrowed space there is reduced blood flow.
- The heart tissue requires oxygen and nutrients to be able to function.
- Restricted blood flow reduces the amount of oxygen delivered.
- When the narrowing becomes severe enough, the oxygen required exceeds the oxygen provided.

You can then go on to explain the symptoms this causes and how it may present:
- Central chest pain
- Pain can also move into the jaw or into the arms (commonly the left arm)
- Shortness of breath
- Nausea and vomiting.

You could then go on to mention some of the potential risk factors.
"A heart attack is more common in..."
- Obesity
- Older age
- Smokers.

If there is any additional information you have picked up through your reading, work experience or education you can mention it, but make sure you have answered the question.

12.5   (T) What do you think is the greatest biological challenge facing medicine today?

Medicine is a constantly changing and evolving field, and that is in part why many feel that a career in healthcare is exciting. There are frequently new discoveries that change the way we think about a disease and its treatment, and so it is important that clinicians are up to date with the basic sciences and research in their specialty.

This question will likely draw many similar answers, and most people will choose either antibiotic resistance or cancer as what they perceive to be the greatest biological challenge we face today. Keep in mind that this question is not looking for a particular answer, but rather one of the most significant problems in medicine, and why you think it is a serious challenge. Thus you are free to choose any reasonable answer; however, it must be a significant current problem in healthcare, and must be something that can be changed or improved, hence the term 'challenge'. As always, it should be accurately backed up by facts. The following structured answer on antibiotic resistance as the greatest biological challenge in medicine shows the following:

- **Background on antibiotic resistance**
- **Problems caused by antibiotic resistance**
- **Current strategies to control antibiotic resistance**
- **Your thoughts on what doctors should be doing to combat this problem.**

"Antibiotic resistance is one of the foremost challenging problems we face in medicine today. In a span of 100 years since the discovery of penicillin, which revolutionised how we treat infectious disease, we have gone full circle and are in danger of losing the efficacy of these important drugs. Every individual at some point in their life will require antibiotic treatment, and over time bacteria have evolved to protect themselves against these drugs, making them ineffective and rendering us susceptible to continued infection.

Resistance on some level has always been plausible, but has been greatly sped up by improper use or over-prescribing. There has been a lot of news brought to the attention of the public about this issue, in order to help inform patients about the importance of taking medications as prescribed. Similarly, healthcare professionals are also being retrained on proper antibiotic guidance. I believe these are stepping stones in the right direction; however, international cooperation is a must. Additionally, there are obstacles that we must overcome, particularly with the issue of funding. Many major pharmaceutical companies have limited interest due to the lack of financial incentive in antibiotic discovery. Currently there has been promising new research into bacteriophages, which are viruses that work against bacteria. However, the working strategy as I understand it is to minimise the need for antibiotics, and proper usage. I think that healthcare professionals lie at the forefront of this battle of resistance prevention, and I'd look forward to learning more about this issue as it progresses."

12.6 *(MMI) You are asked to give a presentation to your fellow medical students on how doctors are regulated in the UK. Explain the advantages and disadvantages of self-regulation in the medical profession. You have 5 minutes to prepare and 7 minutes to present. Please use no resources other than talking. Your interviewer will play the role of the student.*

This question seeks to evaluate your understanding of how doctors are regulated and held accountable for their actions. It also assesses your presentation skills. Basic tips on giving a presentation have already been covered in *Chapter 7*.

The General Medical Council (GMC) regulates UK doctors. The governing body of the GMC is made up of elected doctors, members of the public and academics appointed by medical educational bodies. All doctors working in the UK are required to register with the GMC before starting work and are given a licence to practise.

The main objective of the GMC is to protect the health and safety of the public by ensuring doctors provide a high standard of healthcare and do not cause harm to patients. Failure to do this may result in a GMC investigation. If the doctor is found unfit to practise sanctions, such as suspension or removal of a licence to practise, may be imposed.

The GMC is also responsible for assessing the standards of UK medical education including in medical schools and postgraduate training programmes.

Advantages of self-regulation (i.e. doctors regulating doctors):
- Allows independence for doctors to set their own standards and values.
- The public trust doctors to set and monitor their own professional standards.
- The profession can be trusted to undertake action against individuals when needed.
- There is a high degree of knowledge and skill involved in medicine and non-medical professionals may not be equipped to regulate the actions of medical professionals.

Disadvantages:
- Distrust by some members of the public.
- There may be some inbuilt bias in a profession regulating itself.
- Very heavily regulated with a high paperwork burden for each doctor annually.
- Uncertainty as to how self-regulation will work in the future as NHS care becomes increasingly focused on team working above the individual role of the doctor.

12.7   (T) Should we screen the population for Alzheimer's disease?

A question like this is testing you in several different domains. Firstly it is a good idea to make sure the interviewers are aware that you understand the technical aspects of this question, namely: what is Alzheimer's disease and what is screening? If you are unsure it is far better to be honest and seek some clarification or help, rather than talking confidently about an unrelated topic. Having said that, the interviewers will not expect you to recall a dictionary definition or perhaps even much of the detail, but would hope that you understand **that screening is a process of assessing healthy people with the aim of identifying and treating those that are likely to develop a certain condition or disease.** Again they would expect you to know that Alzheimer's disease is a progressive disease of the brain, generally affecting the elderly, and that it is currently an incurable condition.

Having demonstrated this knowledge one can then tackle the question itself. It is important to convey that you are aware that screening can be an effective means of identifying diseases early on, before they have had a negative impact on the individual. Perhaps one should discuss the economic case for screening – some may feel that society should focus on treating the young rather than on conditions mainly affecting the elderly. This is a highly emotive example, but remember that the interviewers want to see your personality and your passion for medicine. Ensure that you show that you are aware of other opinions, and remain respectful of them – doctors should not be rude or dismissive, even if you do disagree strongly with an alternative point of view.

If time permits you could steer the conversation towards some of the requirements of screening programmes. Show the interview panel that you know that inappropriate screening can lead to more harm than good – is there any benefit in telling a patient they will develop a serious disease if you know there is no treatment available? Is a screening programme acceptable if it is not 100% accurate and you tell some patients that they will develop a nasty disease when they would have remained healthy without your intervention?

12.8   (T) Are you aware of the Hippocratic oath? Briefly, what is it, what does it contain and do you think it is important?

Everyone who wants to study medicine should at least be aware of the Hippocratic oath, historically sworn by doctors at the beginning of their careers.

Named after the famous Greek physician Hippocrates, the oath can be traced back some 2500 years. It contains a series of promises to behave in an ethical manner. Whilst no longer used by most medical schools, many of the principles contained in the oath are acknowledged as being sound guiding ethical and moral principles for a medical career. All doctors must behave with the highest ethical standards, and it is expected that medical students will uphold these values from the very start of their training. A brief understanding of the general thrust of the oath is therefore essential.

Some of the most relevant points of the oath include promises to: share knowledge with colleagues; teach others; treat patients humanely and with respect; remain honest and admit when additional help is required; respect the privacy of the patient; treat the patient as a whole rather than just their disease.

TOP TIP Almost all of these are self-evident and can be remembered, so long as one remembers the gist rather than trying to memorise the exact wording (very few of us are ancient Greek scholars!).

One would be hard pressed to successfully argue against any parts of the Hippocratic oath on principle. The fine details of some parts of the original oath may now be outdated, but they live on in the ethical guidelines required by medical licensing bodies; in the UK this is the General Medical Council (GMC). Before your interview it is advisable to read the GMC's *Good Medical Practice* (2013), as this is essentially an up-to-date and detailed version of the Hippocratic oath that is fit for the modern world.

12.9 (T) How does the role of a doctor differ from that of a nurse practitioner?

This question is seeking to determine what you know about the different roles within medicine. You should start by outlining the role of a doctor:

- Prescribing
- Diagnosing
- Disease management
- Decision making
- Patient care.

You should then give the differences between a doctor and a nurse practitioner. Here are some examples:

- Nurse practitioners are qualified nurses who have undergone further specialist training but do not have a medical degree.
- Nurse practitioners can prescribe; however, what they can prescribe may be limited.

You can then outline any part of medical care that is not provided by a doctor but by another healthcare professional.

- Physiotherapy provided by a physiotherapist
- Washing and dressing provided by a nurse or a health care assistant
- Speech and language therapy provided by a speech and language therapist
- Occupational therapy provides support to enable the person to function as fully as possible.

It is important to say why different people have different roles and why this is important.

- The healthcare team within the NHS is composed of multidisciplinary teams (MDTs).
- This involves a group comprising different staff members, each with different skills that contribute to overall patient care.
- This improves the standard of care.
- For example, a physiotherapist has a different skill set to that of a doctor and as a result they can provide certain specific services that a doctor cannot.

12.10 **(T) Huntington's disease is an inherited condition that damages certain nerve cells in the brain. It is often not apparent until adulthood. The damage gets worse over time, affecting movement and behaviour and ultimately resulting in death. There is no cure. It is diagnosed by genetic testing. Explain to the interviewer the pros and cons of genetic testing being carried out on a patient's 10- and 5-year-old children.**

This question seeks to evaluate your understanding of some of the ethical considerations that need to be taken into account when offering genetic testing.

As Huntington's is an autosomal dominant condition, there is a 50% chance that each child of an affected patient may develop the condition. In the UK anyone with a family history of Huntington's has to be over 18 years of age before they can consent to genetic testing. Because of the implications of a positive test the decision to undergo testing is that of the individual child alone.

Pros of genetic testing:
- They can know for certain.
- If they don't have the faulty gene they don't need to worry about their future.
- If they are affected then they can make plans for the future.
- If they are affected then they may be suitable for a research trial.
- They might want to know as it may impact on their decision to have children themselves.

Cons of genetic testing:
- It may be distressing to live with the knowledge that they will develop Huntington's in the future.
- They might want to enjoy life without knowing, as they might die of another cause before the condition develops.
- One child might be positive and one child negative, causing difficulties in the relationship between siblings.
- It may be difficult to arrange life insurance or a mortgage with a known positive test.
- In a small number of individuals genetic testing cannot give a definitive answer.

12.11 **(MMI) You are a GP seeing Linda, an 89-year-old woman with a recent history of multiple fractures. You diagnose her with a condition called 'osteoporosis', and prescribe her medication to help with the condition. Linda tells you that she has heard some good things about an alternative treatment, which is not available on the NHS. Please explain to Linda that this is not available to her. You will be asked to communicate with an actor in this station who will play Linda. You have 7 minutes to complete the station.**

You will be judged on your ability to show empathy and understanding of the patient's circumstances, while tactfully informing the patient that the NHS does not provide the treatment the patient has requested.

This is a long scenario, so ensure you understand exactly what you have to do before going in and speaking to the patient. It is desirable to have an understanding about osteoporosis, but ultimately not necessary.

- Introduce yourself: "*Hello, my name is Anil, and I am a GP*".
- Confirm the patient's identity and role: "*You must be Linda. I believe you have just been diagnosed with osteoporosis, and want to speak about treatment options?*"
- Listen to the patient: they are likely to tell you about the new medication they would like.
- Fire a warning shot: "*Unfortunately I have some bad news*".
- Inform the patient of your findings empathetically: "*I'm very sorry to say that the treatment you have requested is not available on the NHS.*"
- Take your time when explaining this, ensuring Linda is following the conversation, and judging her reaction.
- Linda may react with confusion or by being quite upset. It is your role to ensure that you are there to support her as she deals with her disappointment.
- Demonstrate empathy: "*I can see that you are feeling upset right now.*"
- Reassure her: "*The standard treatment has been shown to be very effective.*"
- Regardless of what she plans to do next, your role is to support her, and advise her where appropriate.
- This is also an opportunity to demonstrate your knowledge about how drugs are approved within the NHS. You may do this by explaining why the alternative treatment may not be available: "*The treatment you have requested is fairly new, and has not been approved by the National Institute for Health and Care Excellence, which is the organisation that reviews drugs in the UK.*"
- If she is still not convinced, encourage her to seek another professional opinion.

Dealing with patients who want a therapy unavailable on the NHS is a common issue, even one that has been in the news. The NHS is committed to providing the best possible service to the most number of people, but it has its limitations. Understanding and explaining these limitations is important during interview, but also in professional life.

12.12 (T) 'Type 2 diabetes is becoming more common because people are getting fatter.' Is this true?

This question is phrased in a tricky way – essentially it is trying to find out if you know what causes type 2 diabetes mellitus (T2DM). To answer this, you need to draw on your previous scientific knowledge and be able to explain this to the interviewers.

There is no single cause for T2DM – instead, there are various genetic and environmental risk factors that can precipitate its onset in a person. This means that it's difficult to pinpoint one exact cause in an individual – it is most likely the culmination of various factors.

The statement above can be considered somewhat true, as obesity is one of the main modifiable risk factors that can lead to T2DM. In the UK, obesity is on the rise, meaning that more individuals are at risk of developing T2DM. Therefore, the prevalence of diabetes is increasing, i.e. it is becoming more common.

However, obesity is not the only reason T2DM is becoming more common. Other modifiable risk factors, such as smoking and lack of exercise, are also increasing, which, again, is putting more people at risk of developing T2DM.

As well as this, the contributing genetic factors for T2DM are not very well understood. We are aware that it is a polygenic condition (i.e. many different genes can influence its onset) and that there is some kind of hereditary link – however, it is not necessarily true that you will definitely develop T2DM if other members of your family have it.

It's important to stress that T2DM is caused by a combination of lifestyle and genetic factors, so the reason for it becoming more common can't really be picked out as being one specific cause. However, the obesity epidemic is a concern for all doctors, so preventing and managing obesity can be one way to tackle the increase in T2DM.

12.13 **(MMI) You are carrying out a pre-surgery assessment on a patient. She is a heavy smoker. Describe to her the risks of smoking to her health and the outcomes of her surgery. Try to convince her to give up smoking prior to her operation. You have 7 minutes, and will be asked to discuss with an actor who will play the patient.**

Clarify details: The question is purposely vague and encourages candidates to seek more information from the patient.
- When is the operation?
- How long has the patient been smoking?
- How many cigarettes does the patient smoke per day?

Explain the effects of smoking on the patients who undergo surgery:
- Breathing difficulties during and after surgery
- Increased risk of post-operative infection
- Increased risk of clot formation in blood vessels
- Impaired wound healing
- Increased length of stay in hospital.

Offer smoking cessation advice:
- A majority of the research suggests that quitting smoking two or more months prior to surgery provides the most benefit.
- Willpower and determination are the most important aspects to giving up smoking. However, there are ways to help overcome a smoker's addiction to nicotine.
- Nicotine replacement therapy (NRT) can be offered in the form of gum, sprays, patches and lozenges. These can be purchased without a prescription.
- Electronic cigarettes (or e-cigarettes) are designed to mimic the look and feel of cigarettes. They contain a heating element that vaporises a solution to create smoke. In 2015, a study by Public Health England found robust evidence that e-cigarettes are 95% less harmful than tobacco cigarettes. Starter kits for e-cigarettes can be costly (between £15 and £50); however, this is a small amount compared to the lifetime costs of buying cigarettes.
- Stress relief techniques and counselling may also be suggested to the patient.
- Refer the patient for smoking cessation advice – see NHS Choices for further information.

TOP TIP Explore whether the patient has tried to stop smoking in the past and why it was not successful. A strong candidate will exhibit empathy and work with the patient to come up with a plan to quit smoking.

12.14 *(MMI) You are an F1 doctor who is to talk to a patient (who will be played by an actor) who recently had a myocardial infarction (heart attack). After reading the technical information provided on the next page, please explain to your patient what has happened to him. Answer any questions he may have to the best of your ability. You have 7 minutes.*

The accompanying information sheet is full of medical jargon, and it is inappropriate to use these terms with your patient. It is important to (sensitively) assess the extent of your patient's understanding of the topic before explaining it to him. Introduce yourself, confirm your patient's identity and gain permission to discuss events with him before beginning.

"Are you able to tell me, in your own words, what happened to you during your heart attack?"

Enquire as to what exactly he wants to know further to his current knowledge; it may be more or less than you expect. Once you have obtained this information, give him the structure of your explanation to see if he is happy with what you plan to discuss.

He may want to know why one of the vessels supplying his heart became blocked in the first place. Use visual language to make it easier to understand.

"Arteries are tubes; blood flows through the tube to reach the heart at the end. Sometimes, fat begins to line the tube in layers, gradually making the inside of the tube narrower. It's a bit like limescale furring up your plumbing at home. Eventually, the tube may block off completely."

Give information in small chunks, checking your patient is following as you go along. Allow him to ask questions throughout.
"Sometimes, a bit of the fatty material gets exposed when the inside of the artery is damaged. When this happens, sticky clot-forming cells rush to cover the damage, but end up blocking the tube. It could also be that a clot has formed somewhere else in the body, broken off, and travelled to the artery supplying your heart. When the arteries to the heart become blocked, oxygen and nutrients can no longer reach the heart muscle and it becomes damaged. This is what happened to you."

If there is a pen and a sheet of paper available to you, make use of it – visual depictions are often easier to understand than verbal descriptions. Check that the patient has understood the information given to him, if he has any further questions and what sort of support he needs going forward.

"Have I made sense? Is there anything unclear that you would like me to explain again? Thanks for chatting to me today, I hope this has helped."

Myocardial infarction information (for Question 12.14):

A myocardial infarction, commonly known as a "heart attack", occurs when there is an interruption to the blood supply to the heart. The myocardium (heart muscle) becomes starved of oxygen and nutrients. This may lead to ischaemia (a temporary state from which the myocardium can recover) or if it sustained, the myocardium may become infarcted (there is irreversible death of the myocardium in the affected area). There are many different reasons why the arterial supply to the heart may become compromised. A common cause of myocardial infarction is "atherosclerosis" in the arteries supplying the heart: cholesterol aggregations may be deposited in the wall of the artery; these 'atherosclerotic plaques' narrow the diameter of the artery, reducing its elastic capacity and compromising the blood supply to the heart. The plaque may eventually block the artery completely, or it may suddenly rupture. The blood clot that forms around the plaque can also block the artery, as can clots that have travelled to the artery from elsewhere in the body. The symptoms of myocardial infarction include chest pain, nausea and sweating, and a feeling of shortness of breath. Risk factors for atherosclerosis and myocardial infarction include smoking, hypertension (high blood pressure), high cholesterol, diabetes, and having a family history of the condition.

Type 1 diabetes mellitus information (for Question 12.15):

Type 1 diabetes mellitus (T1DM) is an endocrine disorder. The hormone insulin, made by the pancreas and responsible for controlling blood sugar levels, is not produced in someone with T1DM. This is normally down to an autoimmune process, where the immune system acts and destroys the insulin-making cells. If these patients do not inject replacement insulin regularly, they may suffer from hyperglycaemia (having too much glucose in the blood). In the long term, this may result in damage to the arteries. Administering too much insulin can also be a problem for T1DM patients, as blood sugar levels can drop dangerously low. A serious complication of T1DM is diabetic ketoacidosis (DKA), which is when the body tries to form its own energy source as an alternative to glucose, by breaking down body tissues. The resulting 'ketones' are toxic, and may cause the patient to become seriously unwell, marked by a number of things including a high blood sugar. A proportion of T1DM patients are diagnosed for the first time when they have an episode of DKA. Other patients are investigated and diagnosed after reporting symptoms of tiredness, excessive thirst and frequent urination. People with T1DM, particularly if it is poorly controlled, are more prone to infections than people without the disease.

12.15   *(MMI) Please read the information provided (previous page) on Type 1 diabetes mellitus. Pick out the three most relevant 'complications' of diabetes. Explain to the interviewer (without using any medical jargon) why you have chosen these. You have 10 minutes in total: 3 minutes to read the information, and 7 minutes to discuss with the interviewer.*

This question tests your ability to read technical information quickly, pick up on the most salient points and justify your selection. All of the information is about diabetes, so arguably, any three choices could be correct. However, some of the information is just 'interesting' and some is highly relevant.

You may choose to focus on the events that would cause a patient to attend hospital in an emergency, such as severe low or high blood sugar. As these conditions cause a serious decline in the health of the patient and usually require medical management, you would be justified in your choice.

However, the long-term consequences of diabetes – '*damage to the blood vessels*' – give rise to a host of problems for people with diabetes, and for the healthcare professionals involved in their care. Any disruption to the arterial supply of an organ or structure can result in severe disability, such as blindness, or potentially be life-threatening (as in stroke or heart attack). In addition, choosing to highlight that people with T1DM mellitus are more '*prone to infection*' enables you to talk about the risks this poses to the health of the patient beyond those that are immediately evident in the text.

By selecting these pieces of information, you are not only showing you can foresee the clinical consequences of these phenomena, but that you appreciate the fact that the practice of medicine encompasses the lifelong care of patients.

The symptoms of T1DM are an important piece of clinical information. If a person attends a clinic with this group of symptoms, you would expect T1DM to be considered as a potential diagnosis. You may very well pick up on the fact that the patients themselves are (usually) responsible for administering their own insulin, and this is normally done by injection. You could justify this choice to the examiner by explaining that compliance with treatment may vary, potentially giving rise to poor management and therefore complications.

> **TOP TIP** Knowing the role of the pancreas in the disease, the process by which 'ketones' are produced and the fact that T1DM is an 'autoimmune endocrine disorder' are important pieces of information. However, they are full of medical jargon and there are much clearer and relevant complications mentioned in the text.

Chapter 13 | Motivation for medicine

13.1   (T) Do you want to become a doctor to save lives?

This question, if answered well, will differentiate the excellent candidate from the very good. This question both directly challenges a cliché of medicine and indirectly tries to unearth your motivations. Try to avoid a 'yes' or 'no' answer, rather notice the underlying subtext that questions the humanity of doctors. Explore these deeper issues raised by the question.

Of course there are many ways to answer the question – and it may vary depending on what type of specialty attracts you to medicine.

Life and death are important, so be very humble and careful with your choice of words. Do not take these issues lightly:

"It would be an honour to save a life. Doctors do save lives; most commonly those in acute (i.e. emergency or sudden onset) settings. However, I would also see my role as a champion of 'health'. Health has many facets. This may mean me taking on different roles in different circumstances, e.g....:"

- **Listening to my patients.** Sickness can be an emotional time, and being there for my patients at a challenging time will allow me to attempt to affect their mental health in a positive way.
- **Promoting good health.** Lots of illnesses can be avoided. I would encourage those who smoke to stop smoking, and those who have sedentary lifestyles to partake in exercise.
- **Managing long-term illness.** I would see patients with conditions that they have had for a long time. I would aim to manage the condition to prevent further deterioration and to alleviate symptoms.
- **Caring for the dying.** There are circumstances when a patient's care should encompass making them comfortable. Sometimes patients are so ill that we cannot save their lives. In these circumstances ensuring that their symptoms are managed as well as possible is very important.
- **Communicating with patients and family.** Doctors are often called upon to break bad news and explain difficult circumstances. I would aim to do this with great empathy.
- **Leading a team.** I would also be a passionate leader to ensure my team worked with the focus of improving patient care.
- **Researching and teaching.** I would also like to strive to advance medical science and pass on my knowledge to those who are in training.

13.2 (T) Tell me about the traits you saw in the doctors on your work experience.

Work experience gives students an opportunity to understand the day-to-day working life of doctors and assess whether they want to pursue medicine. Whilst on the face of it this question may seem to assess an applicant's motivation to do medicine, it also assesses whether they have a realistic take on life as a doctor and the qualities of a good doctor. Interviewers are not particularly interested in what you did, but rather what you gained and learned as a result of it. Further, they want to ensure you have the necessary characteristics required for a career in medicine.

Don't worry who you have been shadowing. Many students shadow an eminent professor. Whilst this may have been an achievement to organise, it does not necessarily give a realistic approach of the training pathways or the daily life of a doctor, which is what you need to convey.

Rather, there are certain common themes that you should try to bring out. Examples for each will need to be populated from your own work experience, but examples are discussed below. This list is by no way exhaustive, and the desirable attributes of a doctor can all be found via the GMC's document, *Tomorrow's Doctors* (www.gmc-uk.org).

- **Team player:** On one of the days, the FY2 (2nd postgraduate year) on the team called in sick, leaving the team one member short. The registrar (senior trainee), knowing the FY1 (1st postgraduate year) was a newly qualified doctor, would frequently call in between patients during clinic to check on the FY1 and run through patients' management. Shadowing the FY1 at this time, I saw that this gesture gave him great comfort and reassurance on how to treat the patients.
- **Roles in the team:** I noticed how different members in the team had different roles within the team. I saw the junior doctors spent the majority of their time looking after patients and being the main point of contact. However, consultants would split their time variously between the wards, clinics and, for the surgeons, theatres.
- **Teacher:** During ward rounds, the consultant would occasionally stop to teach the junior doctors about the patients. In turn, the junior doctors would also take time out of the ward rounds to explain different issues concerning the patients to me. It was great how the doctors continued to teach at all levels and this is something I feel I would enjoy about working as a doctor.
- **Humility:** I attended a multidisciplinary team meeting during my work experience where complex patients were discussed. It was great to see consultants, experts in their field, openly ask for help from their colleagues, so that their patients would receive the best possible care. It taught me that humility is incredibly important as a doctor, as is the ability to ask for help.

End your answer by summarising the things that you took away from the experience and how that affected your decision to study medicine.

13.3 (T) What work experience have you undertaken and has it helped you make any decisions about your future medical career?

This may be a follow-up question to the previous one, or a stand-alone question. It asks whether your work experience has provided you with some helpful insights into what type of doctor you'd like to be. If you have very little work experience in a hospital or GP surgery you may use examples of alternative work experience (e.g. pharmacy, opticians, physiotherapy, etc.) as supporting reasons for developing an interest in medicine or a particular specialty. If you haven't decided what you would like to do within medicine yet, that is absolutely fine – but you can talk about the aspects of the work experience that you particularly enjoyed.

Read the following example of a poor answer. Despite undertaking a lot of work experience, the candidate has displayed very little insight into a career in medicine and wholly neglected the second part to the question.

"I did work experience at St Somewhere's Hospital. I shadowed a consultant surgeon. I got to watch surgery in theatre, which was daunting at first but I got used to it. Then, I shadowed a GP who was a family friend of my parents. I noticed that it was really difficult for the GP to stick to 10 minutes with each patient. I think I prefer surgery to being a GP. I also spent some time in a local pharmacy but didn't like it."

Furthermore, the candidate has wasted time describing how he/she arranged the work experience in the first place and given unqualified statements about careers as a GP or pharmacist.

Firstly, provide some context to your work experience:
"I shadowed a consultant General Surgeon at a busy university hospital. I saw that he splits his time between clinics, long theatre lists and ward rounds."
The candidate demonstrates understanding of what a surgeon would do on a day-to-day basis.

Secondly, show that you have reflected on aspects of the work experience:
"I witnessed an appendicectomy on a 17-year-old in theatre. Before the operation she was very unwell. The surgeon spoke with empathy to the patient and her parents. After the operation the patient was markedly better."

Finally, relate your answer back to your future medical career:
"This experience has inspired me to seek more information on a career as a surgeon. I feel that a surgical career would be very fulfilling as it allows you to see people get better with something that you have done. However, I am very aware of the demanding nature of the job and career path."

TOP TIP During your work experience, make notes/keep a diary of what you see, any useful hints or tips and how you felt about the experience.

13.4 (T) Do you think medical students experience unique difficulties at university compared to students studying non-vocational courses?

The purpose of this question is to assess how the student will cope at university. There are many additional challenges to studying medicine, particularly in terms of lifestyle and ethical issues that students may encounter during placements. You need to show an understanding of the broader issues affecting medical students and not just the difficulties associated with moving away from home for the first time. This question adds the additional dynamic of comparing the course to other university courses.

Start by appreciating that all students may face difficulties before explaining the differences encountered by studying medicine:
"Starting university is a challenging experience for many students. However, there are often unique [careful with your language here – medical students often feel like they are the hardest-working people on earth, but this should not negate other peoples' problems. Using the word 'unique' makes you sound like you appreciate this, whilst acknowledging that medical courses are indeed challenging] *challenges experienced in studying medicine. These may include...:"*

- Demanding course.
- Acceptance into the medical profession requires students to behave professionally at medical school and in their personal lives.
- Medical students face higher standards of accountability and probity.
- Students will have contact with patients and will need to be presentable and demonstrate the qualities of a doctor during these encounters.
- Students may be faced with ethical situations that they must act on whilst on placement.
- Students may encounter situations whilst on placement that they find emotionally distressing.

Don't forget to finish by acknowledging you hope to thrive despite these challenges:
"I don't approach a medical degree lightly and have given it much consideration. Despite the challenges I have mentioned I believe I am equipped with the skills and experience to be able to thrive even in these challenging situations."

13.5 (T) What do you understand by the term 'lifelong learning'?

This is an important question and assesses if you have done background research before deciding to embark on a career in medicine.

Remember a career in medicine involves lifelong learning! You cannot simply stop after five or six years of medical school.

Start by defining the statement. For example:
"For me lifelong learning means learning and acquiring new knowledge – not just from a formal teaching environment but from many other sources. This learning carries on after university and continues throughout your career."

Next explain what lifelong learning means in medicine. For example:
"In the medical field lifelong learning means constantly learning and updating your knowledge after you graduate from medical school. It involves learning each time you see a patient or encounter a new disease or disorder. From what I witnessed during my work experience, junior doctors do get some formal teaching each week from the consultants. Lifelong learning also involves studying for your postgraduate membership exams and attending medical conferences and reading medical journals to keep up to date."

Next explain why lifelong learning is important.

It is important because:
- Medicine is evidence-based so doctors need to learn and keep up with the latest knowledge to provide safe, effective medical care.
- Treatments and management protocols that you learn in medical school or as a junior doctor may be very outdated when you get to a senior level. This means there is no alternative but for doctors to keep updating their practice.

To answer the question effectively, follow these steps:
- Define in your own words what lifelong learning is.
- Relate it to medicine.
- Explain why it is important.
- State that you are looking forward to lifelong learning and updating your knowledge constantly to provide safe effective care for your future patients.

13.6   (T) What led you to pursue a career in medicine?

Whilst this is a predictable question, try not to sound over-rehearsed.

It is a common question that most applicants are asked during interview, and one question that most people have prepared an answer for. While it is important to be prepared and to expect this question, be careful not to memorise a long, generic answer and sound rehearsed. This will not come across well, especially as interviewers will have heard hundreds of similar answers! This is an opportunity for you to be honest about how you came to the decision of wanting to be a doctor, and to show the panel just how passionate you are!

Talk about your experiences. Was it an interest in science that sparked your interest?

Did you explore many options before settling on medicine? This doesn't make you any less committed than someone else and may even make your decision come across as very considered. If this is the case you can even talk about work experience you've had in other careers and why you preferred medicine.

Drawing upon your experiences will make your answer automatically more spontaneous and you will come across as being genuinely enthusiastic.

Perhaps there was a particular moment where you saw doctors in action? Perhaps you or a family member had to go to hospital and the experience inspired you? Or maybe you simply have medicine as a logical option due to your love of sciences and passion for interaction with people.

Back up your answer with some of your work experiences:
Next show that you have put a lot of thought into pursuing medicine. Talk about how you spent that week during your holidays at a GP surgery or shadowing a hospital doctor. You need to give some evidence of your dedication to studying medicine.

13.7 (T) Applicants to medical school are well qualified and highly motivated. Being a doctor will not make you rich; why not choose to pursue a far better paid career in the City?

Aside from the obvious answer that there's more to life than money, this is the time to focus on the myriad of positives a medical career brings. It is perhaps helpful to address the issue of money first in order that it does not become the 'elephant in the room' – whilst one should not pursue a medical career to get rich, it will provide a stable and comfortable income.

There are a great number of reasons that make a medical career more tempting than a lucrative career in City finance for many, particularly the aspiring medical student. Whilst everyone is bound to provide a different list there are several that must surely be hard to ignore. Life as a doctor brings variety – different conditions affecting different people in different ways.

Another oft-cited selling point is altruism – spending your time attempting to improve your patients' lives is truly rewarding. The opportunity to travel is also often given to adventurous young medics; medicine crosses borders and breaks down barriers. As a doctor trained in a well-respected healthcare system one is able to travel almost anywhere on the planet; indeed one could even carve out a niche working under the waves or in space – wherever humans go, medical expertise is required.

Medicine is a scientific discipline and as such changes and evolves, as the underlying science becomes better understood. Working in such a fluid field, even having the power to shape the direction a given field takes, is particularly tempting to some aspiring clinical researchers.

13.8   (T) Why don't you want to become a nurse instead?

This can be a challenging question to answer without inadvertently being dismissive of an entire highly skilled profession when in the pressure of an interview situation. There are of course differences between a career in nursing and a career in medicine. Ensure you emphasise these as *differences* rather than any suggestion that a medical career is superior to a nursing career. Optimal patient care depends on each member of the multidisciplinary team bringing something slightly different to the table, whilst working together and treating each other with respect.

Drawing the line between what doctors and nurses do is increasingly difficult, with some nurses now licensed to prescribe, to order investigations and carry out complex procedures – a stereotype of nurses cleaning patients while doctors attend to the patient's malady is even more outdated than ever before.

The ultimate responsibility for a patient in hospital lies with the consultant they are admitted under – in this way those in medicine are required to develop management skills and are expected to lead a team. Many nurses also take on management roles, but this is often more of a choice than an expectation. If one has a real desire to train as a surgeon then it is of course essential to train as a doctor; nurses may train to perform complex procedures but their practice is also under the supervision of a consultant.

This question could either be asked by itself or, more likely, as an extension to other interview questions such as:

- Why do you want to be a doctor? (If this has not already been asked then ensure you cover your reasons for choosing medicine in your answer.)
- What is the role of a nurse/nurse practitioner?
- How do the roles of doctors and nurses differ?
- What are the component team members of the 'multidisciplinary team'?

13.9 (T) Are there any clinicians who have inspired you to study medicine and become a doctor?

Whilst this is clearly a highly personal question, and should be answered as such, there are several points that it would be beneficial to consider:

- What did they do that made them stand out?
- How did they inspire you?
- Was it a doctor, nurse or other healthcare professional that made the difference?

Discuss this topic with friends or family – even if they aren't interested in a medical career themselves, it is highly likely that they will recognise and admire some of the characteristics that various ethical codes and oaths seek to uphold: honesty, integrity and excellent communication. People expect all their doctors to possess the required knowledge, although nobody can know everything, so the real onus on healthcare professionals is to communicate well, to be honest and to behave with integrity. Patients consistently rate doctors who communicate effectively better than those who cannot maintain an effective doctor–patient relationship.

It would certainly be worth considering if you have ever met any medical professionals who you felt did not meet the required standard. In what way did they fail to perform? How would you ensure you don't make the same mistakes? When you are chief of department or clinical director how would you lead by example and ensure your team all meet your high standards?

13.10 (T) If you are unsuccessful in your application for medicine, what will you do next?

This question seeks to establish your dedication to medicine. Medical schools are looking for candidates who are sure that medicine is definitely what they want to do. Your answer should be personal to you but should also demonstrate your commitment to the career choice. It is important to show an understanding of how competitive medicine is and that you are aware that there is a possibility that you will not be successful in your application.

You can start your answer by stating what your plan would be if you are unsuccessful, and explaining your reasons. The answer will depend on your situation: whether you are applying while still studying for A levels, after a gap year or after graduating.

Some of the options available are:
*   To reapply to study medicine. If an applicant is not successful on their first application, this does not mean he or she could never be a good doctor. There are many applicants competing for one place and all will have very similar qualities. If this is your answer, you should explain what you would do between applications that would make you a better candidate. e.g. more work experience in a care home or hospital.
*   To go to university and study a different course. This may be because you think that if you are unsuccessful it was not meant to be. Be careful about this answer as this may show the interviewers you aren't committed. You must explain why.
*   To study another course and apply for graduate entry. You need to demonstrate understanding by stating the advantages and disadvantages of applying for graduate entry, e.g. finances and fierce competition.

You could then finish the question by summarising what would make you a good medical student and why you think you should be successful in this application. While this is not asked of you in the question, it gives you the opportunity to demonstrate why you are an excellent candidate. An example is:
"This is not a decision I have taken lightly; I have researched what it takes to become a doctor and my work experience to date has shown me that this is something I definitely want to do. I believe that my 'experiences and qualifications' make me a competitive candidate and I hope that you will consider me to be ready for a place in this academic year."

13.11 (T) Everyone in medical school will have been top of their class during their school life. How will you continue to stay motivated in medical school if you are no longer at the top of the peer group?

This question is assessing your ability to cope in a competitive environment and to demonstrate that you are capable of motivating yourself.

It may be considered naïve if you fail to acknowledge that you may no longer be top of the class, as all applicants have the same high standards placed on them for medical school entry and will all have very high grades. Of course, one student will be at the top but to say that you will be that student without any experience of the course itself will not be taken well and may make you come across as arrogant. This doesn't mean that you should undersell yourself but be careful in your phrasing.

You should start by explaining that you have an understanding of the medical school environment:
- Medical school is very competitive.
- All students have very similar and high level qualifications.
- The work is very different from what you will have done previously.
- The bar is set very high in medical exams and the pass mark is often higher than those in other subjects: no one wants a doctor who only knows 40% of what they should know!

You should then describe what you would do to ensure you meet your 'full potential':
- Aim to understand at an early stage what the best method of learning is for you.
- Commit to extra reading as necessary.
- Work with other medical students to share ideas.
- Gain the help of a senior member of staff at the university at an early stage, should you begin to struggle.
- Put your learning in context – go to see patients with the condition you are learning about.

You could give an example of a situation when you were in a highly competitive situation, and how you handled it:
- If you participate in a sports team, in a high level competition where you weren't the winner.
- If you were not top of the class in a particular subject at A level, etc.

You can finish with a statement explaining that you realise the importance of your mental wellbeing and would spend time unwinding, playing sport or socialising with friends, perhaps as a reward for a busy working week.

13.12 (T) It is clear from your personal statement that you enjoy science – why not become a scientist?

This is a common question, with a fairly straightforward answer. It is very similar to the *"If you want to care for people, why not be a nurse?"* question.

The key to answering the question is to make it personal, and refer to your work experiences while doing so.

A model answer may be:

- **Address the fact that you enjoy science**: *"I do enjoy science; it is for this reason that I picked biology and chemistry to study in my A levels."*
- In their initial years, medical students study almost purely science. Even in career progression, one should remain up to date on the research around one's specialty.
- Show that you have contemplated this question yourself: *"I thought I might enjoy being a scientist, so I spoke to a researcher at my local university about his experiences and his job."*
- Show your **understanding** of the career: *"From what I understood, there is very little, if any, patient contact as a scientist."*
- Tie in your work **experience**: *"When I shadowed a gynaecologist, I really enjoyed speaking to patients and liked the idea of helping them through their problems."*
- Come to a **conclusion**: *"While I enjoy science, I also enjoy patient contact. I think that would give me a lot of satisfaction in my career. It is for this reason that I think I would be better suited to a career as a doctor than a scientist."*

13.13 (T) What steps have you taken in the past to make sure that medicine is the right career for you?

Every year, each medical school gets many more applicants than they have places and to try to narrow down their choices the interviewers want to find out if you have the drive to continue in medicine or if you'll potentially give up at some point. This question is a really good opportunity to go through important parts of your personal statement. The interviewers want to know what experiences you've had in the past or what you've done to find out if medicine is a viable career for you.

Talking about your work experience will form a large part of your answer – try to explain how it prepared you for a potential medical career. What did you do, when and where? Was it primary or secondary care? How did it feel talking to patients or getting to listen to consultations? You can really elaborate on points that you've made in your personal statement, as chances are, you've had to be quite succinct when writing it! Reflecting on your patient contact time and your experiences of a medical environment will show the interviewers that you're serious about wanting to follow medicine. For instance:

"I shadowed a local GP for a week to try and gain some insight into the field. Although I have never previously considered a career in primary care, this work experience was invaluable to me, as I really came to appreciate the ongoing and holistic care that patients receive from GPs. It also gave me further understanding of the role of a GP – as well as consultations, GPs work a lot behind the scenes, including checking prescriptions, ensuring safeguarding and so much more. Although this seemed like a lot of work, it seemed to be a rewarding career and one that I feel I have the determination to pursue..."

Although it's not necessarily an advantage to know someone or have a family member in medicine, you should try to make the most of it if you do. Family members, especially, will give you a realistic insight into the field and you can really see how medicine affects the rest of an individual's life.

You can also use examples of various skills you've shown in the past to back up why medicine is the career for you. This includes things like dedication, good time management and effective communication skills. These are all important and necessary attributes for a good doctor so if you've demonstrated these in the past, the interviewers will be assured that you have what it takes, e.g.

"Over the past two years, I have been volunteering at a local nursing home once a week. My role involves assistance at meal times and handing out cups of tea to residents. Although this may seem minor to some, I really enjoy spending time with the elderly residents and we all look forward to this weekly slot. It also shows that I am motivated to work in the healthcare field."

Chapter 14 |
National Health Service (NHS) questions

14.1 (T) What do you think a 'multidisciplinary team' (MDT) is and why is it important in healthcare?

This question seeks to evaluate your understanding of teamwork in healthcare, which is key to how the NHS works.

A multidisciplinary team is a group of professionals who work together to help provide the best pathway of diagnosis and treatment for a patient.

It would help to understand what an MDT is. It depends on why the team exists as to who is in it, but it can often comprise:
- Medical doctors e.g. respiratory doctors if a lung MDT, gastroenterologists if for a bowel disease, oncologists if for cancer
- Surgeons
- Doctors with a specialist skill e.g. psychiatrists if a mental health MDT, paediatricians if a children's MDT
- Physiotherapists
- Radiologists
- Occupational therapists
- Dieticians
- Pathologists

It meets to discuss patient cases and uses available information such as blood results, the patient's history, X–rays and tissue sample results.

You should also give a statement about why teamwork in this setting is important:
- Brings together a breadth of skill
- Facilitates discussion as to the best treatment options
- Provides an efficient way of gaining the opinions of multiple professionals.

14.2   (T) What is the role of a 'consultant'?

This question serves as an excellent opportunity to showcase your up-to-date knowledge on the ever-changing NHS.

There are five main roles of a consultant:

1. A consultant is a specialist in their area. Complicated or rare cases which need specialist input are referred to consultants. They may even lead research groups and be involved in development of new treatments.

2. Consultants are educators. They spend large amounts of time teaching students, junior doctors, allied healthcare professionals, the public and patients.

3. Consultants are leaders both for the service they provide and of the healthcare service. As experts, their opinion is often sought in public health initiatives and in planning the future of the NHS.

4. Consultants are patient advocates. Consultants have influence and should use this to cater to the evolving needs of patients and to break down barriers to improved patient care.

5. Above all, consultants are often still practising frontline doctors and make decisions on patient care and are a point of contact for advice for more junior colleagues.

The role of consultants continues to evolve, and the health service is moving towards a more 'consultant-led' service. This means that more consultant time will be spent on frontline patient care in the future. This may warrant a follow-up question from the interviewer at this stage about whether you think this is a good idea. Be prepared with a few pros and cons:

Pros:
- More timely decision making for patients
- Urgent expert opinions can be sought easily.

Cons:
- Less time may be spent on innovation and medical breakthroughs
- Less time spent on leadership and management, meaning more non-clinicians making strategic decisions.

14.3 (T) Tell us about some of the changes the NHS has recently gone through.

The NHS has gone through huge changes, making the answer to this question vast. Acknowledge this in your answer.

Your answer should include at least three or four important changes, with two more in your mind if pressed for more. Briefly explain the changes in a couple of sentences and pick one to discuss in detail, providing a balanced argument for and against the change.

Some changes to the NHS are outlined in the Department of Health White Paper, *Equity and Excellence* (2010):
www.gov.uk/government/uploads/system/uploads/attachment_data/file/213823/dh_117794.pdf

Commentary may be found on the website of the health think-tank King's Fund:
www.kingsfund.org.uk/topics/nhs-reform/nhs-white-paper

- **Abolishment of Primary Care Trusts (PCTs)**

The 152 PCTs responsible for deciding on funding for primary, secondary and community health services were abolished in 2013 under the Health and Social Care Act 2012 and 'Clinical Commissioning Groups' were introduced instead.

- **Introduction of Clinical Commissioning Groups (CCGs)**

CCGs are groups of, primarily, GPs, but can also contain secondary care doctors, allied health professionals and lay people, who together commission or buy healthcare services.

- **Opening NHS market to increased competition from independent companies**

This is an effort to streamline the NHS and gain the best value for money. Others see it as a form of privatisation.

- **New regulatory body: Care Quality Commission (CQC)**

Replaces a number of quality control bodies. CQC oversees all healthcare institutions providing care under the NHS (including private companies). It performs regular inspections of hospitals and can make recommendations on their performance.

- **Closer relationship between health, social care and mental healthcare**

There is an initiative to ringfence mental health funds and to build bridges between health and social care, both of which are intrinsically linked. Increased success in social care in turn reduces the healthcare and mental health burden.

- **Shift to providing more care in the community**

In an effort to combat increased hospital admissions, especially via Emergency Departments, increasingly complex care is being provided in patients' homes and GP surgeries.

14.4 (T) How much does the NHS cost each year, what is the biggest expenditure and how is it funded?

This question is assessing whether you understand the infrastructure that you will be working in. It is important to understand the NHS and to take an active role in keeping up to date with the changes, as they will directly affect the capacity in which you will work. Whilst you may not be expected to be able to rattle off the exact figures it would be important to be realistic (i.e. it will be in the billions of pounds – certainly not millions!).

It is also important to at least have a grasp of where the NHS may be going politically, e.g. have you read about how much the current government intends to invest in the NHS? If not, have a quick read online now!

Open with a line such as:
"The NHS costs a significant sum of money each year. Whilst I am unsure [or if you are sure – say so!] of the exact figure it will be in the tens or hundreds of billion pounds per year."

You can then demonstrate your wider understanding of the costs and where they are likely to head:
"I realise that there are a number of factors influencing healthcare costs. These include the ageing population and greater variety of procedures/drugs available on the NHS. This will lead to increasing costs of healthcare. This is at a time when other public services are undergoing budget cuts, which may have an impact on the NHS."

You can really show off if you know the facts:
- In 2014/2015 the NHS net expenditure (resource plus capital, minus depreciation) was approximately £114 billion. The planned expenditure for 2015/2016 is approximately £117 billion.
- The biggest expenditure is staff salaries, comprising approximately two thirds of the total NHS budget.
- The NHS is funded by taxation.

To keep up to date with the statistics the NHS confederation site is a good place to find clear information: www.nhsconfed.org/resources/key-statistics-on-the-nhs

14.5 (T) What is your understanding of the biggest challenge the NHS currently faces?

The NHS and health economy is always a topical issue in the UK, so it will be no news to you that the NHS is currently facing several challenges, particularly the issue of rising costs of healthcare. During medical school, students will be taught about basic health economics and have lectures on the NHS. Interviewers who ask this question will be interested to know how engaged you are with the healthcare sector, not just medicine as a discipline. There is no absolute right or wrong answer – but some challenges the NHS faces are not specific but seen in any universal healthcare system, and so should not be chosen for your answer. A good working knowledge of the NHS and how services are funded and delivered is paramount.

The example answer below addresses the issue of an ageing population, and its effect on the rising costs of the NHS. You should aim to answer this question with:

Background:
"The UK has an ageing population, who are increasingly suffering from long-term (or 'chronic') diseases and this can cause significant challenges to healthcare delivery."

The challenge to healthcare delivery and why it is significant:
"An ageing population is significant because patients are living longer with more complex conditions, which may require frequent hospital admissions or long courses of expensive medication. This causes costs of healthcare to rise.

In addition, an ageing population means that a smaller proportion of people are contributing financially to the NHS as a publicly funded system."

A solution to address the challenge:
"Putting more resources into preventing illness before it even starts could alleviate the problem. This means more 'public health' measures such as encouraging healthy eating and exercise. More resources for community care may result in less hospital care being required."

Why it is an important issue for doctors:
"An ageing population usually results in patients with multiple conditions all at once, which can make diagnosis and treatment difficult decision-making processes. In addition, to conserve resources in a publicly funded system doctors may be required to reorganise the way healthcare is provided, and to move more services into the community."

14.6 (T) How do politics affect the way the NHS is run? Do you think there is too much political intervention in the NHS?

When answering this question, maintain an unbiased view that is based on facts, and not one based on your particular political position. This may be a difficult question to tackle, and it is important that you read up on the different political parties in the UK, and what their stance on the NHS is and has been over the last ten years (particularly in the last general election). As the NHS is a publicly funded institution, and we live in a democratic country whereby the public determine the politicians in charge, it is reasonable to expect a certain level of political power over the NHS. It is when the NHS is used purely for political gain that it becomes problematic, and the public and profession should lobby politicians in charge, so that the direction the NHS takes is democratic. Satisfaction with the NHS has also taken distinct trends over time, depending on the political party in government.

A sample discussion point on the interaction between politics and the NHS is outlined below:

"As our health service is publicly funded, it is expected that there will be public involvement through the politicians elected to government. However, consultation with stakeholders is vital to ensure the national system works well with the government. An example of this includes the announcement about the establishment of a 7-day NHS service in 2015. Some news outlets reported that healthcare workers were offended by the Health Secretary's comments at the time, and the medical staff wanted to see further evidence that the changes would be for the better. The relationship between the two parties broke down and doctors took part in strike action following the result of a ballot by the British Medical Association.

Had the situation been handled differently, perhaps by both parties, the situation would have been different. This highlights that politics can hugely affect the NHS."

As in the above answer, try to keep in mind the following points when formulating your response:
- Unbiased and apolitical – do not swing towards one political party or another.
- Expand on how political intervention affects the public who use it and the workers who provide the service.

14.7 (T) The NHS has been described as 'the envy of the world'. How does it differ from publicly funded healthcare systems in other parts of the world?

A good working knowledge of different healthcare models in developed countries helps immensely with this question, so it will require a fair amount of background reading. Specifically, the question addresses the performance of the NHS against other similar publicly funded services, such as the universal healthcare sector in Canada. One particular report, *Mirror, Mirror on The Wall* by The Commonwealth Fund, is a highly recommended read as it places the NHS ahead of eleven other healthcare systems in the world for multiple parameters. Knowing the strengths of the NHS is as important as knowing the weaknesses, as you want your answer to be balanced and thorough.

You can approach this question by touching on the following points:
- **NHS performance in healthcare delivery and cost efficiency**
  - The NHS was ranked in first place in terms of the following patient care metrics: effective care, safe care, patient–centred care and coordinated care. It also ranked first in terms of overall efficiency, indicating that the NHS is ahead of countries such as Canada, France and Germany in these parameters of effective care delivery. The NHS is also one of the most cost-efficient systems.
- **Cancer diagnosis and treatment performance**
  - Cancer is one of the leading causes of mortality worldwide, and since an effective cure doesn't exist for many types of cancer, the speed at which we diagnose cancer makes a great amount of difference to patient survival. This is one of the issues that are often sensationally highlighted in the media, as the UK currently lags behind the rest of Europe in cancer survival, according to some sources.
- **Coverage offered in the NHS vs. other systems**
  - Many healthcare systems that are universal do not provide as widespread coverage as the NHS. Whereas in the UK, patients pay only a prescription dispensing charge (in England) per drug, other countries with universal healthcare such as Canada require patients to pay for the entire cost of the drug or otherwise be covered by drug insurance (through employment or private insurance). This is a massive strength for the NHS, and a good point to highlight in your answer.

Recommended reading:
The Commonwealth Fund (2014). *Mirror, Mirror on the Wall*. Available at: www.commonwealthfund.org/publications/fund–reports/2014/jun/mirror-mirror

14.8 (T) What do you think are the similarities and differences between a hospital in the UK and one in a developing country?

Talk about your experiences

If you have been fortunate enough to do work experience in a developing country you should link it to this question. Talk about anything you experienced during your time there. Even if you have no first-hand experience of a hospital in a developing country you can make an educated guess.

Similarities:

- Doctors and healthcare professionals all work together as a team with the aim of helping patients get better.
- Unwell patients are in an unfamiliar environment, and are therefore some of the most vulnerable members of society.
- Doctors and nurses help to support patients during difficult times.

Differences:

- Resource limitations in developing countries may lead to doctors relying heavily on their clinical skills to form management plans. They may not have access to expensive tests such as MRI scans, etc.
- Lack of trained healthcare staff in more rural areas may mean more lay members of the community helping in the hospital than in resource-rich settings.
- Patients in resource-rich areas are more likely to suffer from heart disease and other lifestyle-related illnesses, whereas those in a resource-poor country are likely to have more acute infections.
- In resource-poor settings there may be lack of access to vaccinations and other preventative measures.

There are many other similarities and differences that you could talk about. If you are struggling to find things, think about what is universal in healthcare, and what can be affected by factors such as funding, demographics, and resources.

Finishing the question

You can mention that we are incredibly fortunate to have a healthcare system that provides free healthcare to all at the point of delivery, and briefly summarise your key points.

You could finish with a sentence that shows that hospitals in both settings have ultimately the same goal: to put patients at the heart of everything they do.

14.9   (T) Discuss the advantages and disadvantages of the privatisation of the NHS.

This is a very hot topic, and therefore a question could easily come up in your interview. You should have a reasonable understanding of the current political agendas, and be able to discuss them if asked.

Start off the answer by explaining the current situation in the NHS

It is important to understand what the question means by 'privatisation'. The privatisation of the NHS does not necessarily mean a US-style system where healthcare is funded by private insurance, although you may wish to touch on the advantages and disadvantages of such a system.

In the NHS private companies already contribute to care in various ways – either by running entire hospitals and GP practices or by providing services within an NHS hospital e.g. running the canteen, providing cleaning services or sterilising the theatre equipment.

Next, be able to talk about the key advantages and disadvantages. There may be several other points you would like to talk about:

Advantages:

- Private companies are an additional way in which patients can be treated and as such, result in an increase in patient choice.
- NHS hospitals can outsource, as necessary, some of their care to private units to keep waiting times down for patients.
- The private system may be more efficient, given that profit-making firms have a drive to ensure costs remain low.

Disadvantages:

- Cherry-picking of cases by the private sector may lead to only the sicker (and potentially less 'profitable') patients being left in the NHS, affecting the NHS hospitals' incomes.
- Trainees, who are based in NHS hospitals, may not see the 'routine' cases, negatively affecting their learning experience.
- It may result in corners being cut by private firms in order to ensure profits remain high.

Conclude by giving your opinion on the matter, based on the well-balanced points you have talked about, making sure you have given reasonable evidence for your view.

14.10   (T) Tell me what you know about the Francis report/ Mid Staffordshire inquiry. What implications will it have for the NHS in the future?

The Mid Staffordshire Inquiry was a public inquiry, led by Robert Francis, a barrister. It was launched as a response to a number of earlier inquiries that had identified a higher than expected mortality rate in Stafford Hospital, under the management of the Mid Staffordshire Trust. This wide-ranging enquiry reported in February 2013, making 290 recommendations. A summary of the report can be found at the link below: www.gov.uk/government/uploads/system/uploads/attachment_data/file/279124/0947.pdf

This question aims to assess if you have been keeping yourself up to date with major news stories related to health, as well as to judge if you understand the implications of a report as significant as the Francis report.

In answering questions such as this, it is always better to read around the subject, from a number of different sources (including the one above) and speak freely about it during the interview, as a pre-learned answer may sound rehearsed. However, an example is given below for reference.

It is best to start the answer with a brief description of the Francis report, demonstrating you know more about the facts surrounding the report than was revealed in the question.

"The Francis report was the report of a public inquiry into failings in patient care in Stafford Hospital, part of the Mid Staffordshire NHS Trust. It was commissioned in response to previous reports that suggested a high number of avoidable deaths and to the complaints of patients' relatives."

Following this, you should describe some of the key failings identified in the inquiry, as well as point out the key recommendations.

"The inquiry identified a number of issues in the way the hospital was being run, not least of which was the less-than-open culture when mistakes were made. Furthermore, the report identified that the management may have put financial concerns ahead of concerns about staffing levels. The report had 290 recommendations in all, with a key recommendation being that a culture of openness and transparency should predominate in all NHS trusts, with people encouraged to highlight poor practice, so that problems such as those that were happening in Stafford Hospital could be identified and dealt with much earlier. This report has already had an impact on NHS policy, with all hospitals now having to publish their staffing levels, as well as the percentage of shifts that meet safe staffing levels."

14.11 **(MMI) You are a medical student coming to the end of the first week of your placement in general surgery. There are numerous posters in the ward providing hand washing instructions that you have been following dutifully. The ward round in the morning is very busy and you have noticed that the consultant is not consistently washing his hands between seeing patients. Does this matter? Does this mean that it is OK for you not to wash your hands? Do you say anything? Please outline your answer to the interviewer. You have 5 minutes to do so.**

This question is testing your ethics and ability to raise difficult conversations with your seniors that are necessary to ensure good patient care.

Hand washing and infection control are extremely important in the healthcare setting as they prevent the transmission of bacteria and pathogens between patients. Every year over 300 000 patients in England acquire a healthcare-associated infection.

All staff should wash their hands:
- **Before touching a patient**
- **Before an aseptic task**
- **After exposure to bodily fluids**
- **After patient contact**
- **After contact with a patient's surroundings**.

It is the responsibility of all staff to ensure that everyone is compliant. You should continue to wash your hands and encourage others to do so.

You also have a duty of care to the patients that you are seeing and will need to address the issue that your consultant is not washing his hands. This can be very difficult due to the hierarchical nature of medicine and it can be very difficult to reproach someone in a much senior position.

What course of action you take will depend on your confidence level as well as your relationship with your consultant. You might feel more comfortable discussing your concerns with another member of staff such as the ward sister who will be able to remind your consultant.

14.12 **(MMI) A political party has declared that it would pay medical students around £10 000 during their studies for committing to go into a specialty that is currently undersubscribed (e.g. emergency or elderly medicine, general practice). What do you think are the pros and cons of this strategy? You have 7 minutes to discuss your views with the interviewer.**

It is worth keeping an eye on the news as it is frequently a topic of discussion in interviews. It can help gauge a candidate's interest in medicine and demonstrates an awareness of current affairs. It is very possible that you may be asked about an article you have not seen. In this case it is perfectly acceptable to say that you have not read/seen that article *"but that it sounds very interesting"*. Even if you haven't heard about the article before, you may still be asked your opinion about the subject. Below is a basic structure for answering such a question:

If you have read the article, give a brief summary of the article before starting. This has two functions: firstly, it proves that you have indeed read the article and secondly, it shows that you can effectively summarise it.

If you have not read the article, you can start with something like this: *"I haven't read that article but it sounds like something I would like to read about. Without seeing the article myself it might be difficult to give a full and informed answer, but based on the information given..."*

Below are some pros and cons of the above proposal.

Pros:
- Will help to boost numbers of doctors in undersubscribed specialties
- Will help to address the needs of future patients
- Provides medical students with financial support for their studies, making it less likely for students to sacrifice studying time to part-time jobs
- Increases interest in those specialties.

Cons:
- Forces students to commit to a specialty too early in their career when they have little experience of other job roles
- Students may ultimately be forced into a career they no longer want to do, leading to an unmotivated workforce or poor staff retention
- Monetary incentives are disproportionately more likely to attract those students who are less well off rather than those who may be best suited
- Although £10 000 is a lot of money to a student, it is a small amount compared to the rest of a working career
- The money used to fund the scheme may deprive other areas of the NHS.

Once you have presented arguments from both sides, try to conclude with a single sentence. E.g. *"Overall, I feel that although the scheme is trying to address a significant problem, this proposal appears to target less wealthy students, potentially 'forcing' them into careers before they have the ability to make an informed choice."*

14.13   *(MMI) You are shadowing a consultant who tells you that the NHS is failing and privatisation is not only inevitable, but also necessary. Discuss your own views with the consultant. You will be asked to communicate with an actor in this station. You have 7 minutes to complete the station.*

This station is testing your basic knowledge about the NHS and its future, as well as your ability to form an opinion and argue your case. Your opinion can swing towards privatisation or the NHS – as long as you are aware of the arguments on both sides.

To tackle the conversation you should:

- **Introduce yourself:** *"Hello, my name is Jenny and I am a first-year medical student. Can I check your name please?"*
- **Outline the conversation:** *"I believe you wanted to discuss privatisation and the NHS?"*
- **State your stance on the topic whilst demonstrating that you appreciate their point of view:** *"I appreciate the arguments you have given about privatisation although unfortunately I disagree with the view that the NHS is failing, and privatisation is necessary".*
- **State an argument in favour of your stance:** *"The NHS has faced substantial financial challenges in the past, and has managed to overcome these."*
- **Back this statement up with an example if possible:** *"For example, in 1987, the NHS was plunged into the worst financial crisis of its history. In response, in 1991, the 'internal market' for the NHS was established."*
- **Provide between one and three considered points for your argument and explain them.**
- **Provide one or two points for the other side of the argument, to show your ability to balance an argument:** *"However, I understand that privatisation may be thought to reduce waiting times, and increase the efficiency of the healthcare system."*
- **Reiterate your opinion to close your argument:** *"Despite the factors against the continuation of the NHS, I believe providing healthcare free at the point of contact is remarkable, and a challenge that many countries struggle to accomplish. For this reason, I believe that the NHS is worth holding on to."*

14.14 (T) Doctors don't wear white coats any more. What are the pros and cons of doctors wearing white coats?

In the UK, the doctor's white coat was phased out in the early 2000s, yet it had been the standard attire for the profession for over 150 years. In many other countries around the world, it is still worn by medics. In your answer, think about why the white coat lasted for so long and also the reasons why it might have been replaced in the UK.

One of the big advantages of white coats is that they are easily recognisable. Everyone, staff and patients, is aware that the individual wearing the white coat is a doctor. In the same way that nurses are asked to wear the same colour tunics/dresses, the white coat was a similar 'uniform' for doctors. The white coat also makes it easier for all doctors to appear smart and professional. You can incorporate these points with some of your own personal experiences, e.g.:

"I think one of the great advantages of doctors wearing the white coat was that it was probably easier for everyone to identify who they were. At times while on work experience, I struggled to identify which staff members were doctors, especially if their ID badges weren't very obviously displayed. The white coat was probably really helpful in this respect."

Some studies have shown that a large number of patients actually prefer their doctors to be wearing white coats – this is probably truer in the older generation, who might like the formality of the doctor–patient relationship.

However, in the same way, the white coat may actually act as a psychological barrier between doctors and others around them. Patients, in particular, might find it harder to disclose information or it may have other adverse effects on consultations, e.g. 'white coat hypertension'.

One of the main reasons white coats were banned in the UK was for infection prevention issues. As well as not adhering to the 'bare below the elbows' policy that is in place in most UK hospitals, white coats weren't being washed and cleaned as often as was necessary, so they were potentially cross-infecting patients. You can really emphasise the point of patient safety with this argument against white coats.

"However, white coats were found to be an infection risk, as they were harbouring micro-organisms and carrying disease from one patient to the next when they were seen by the doctor. The white coat, then, can potentially compromise patient safety, as it could lead to patients contracting extra, avoidable diseases. Ensuring patient safety is one of the main duties of a doctor, so this is one of the white coat's biggest disadvantages."

14.15 **(MMI) Some people are of the view that deterrent fees (a small charge, which everyone who visits the GP would have to pay) would be an effective way to control health costs. You are a local GP and have been asked to discuss this concept with a Department of Health finance executive. You will be asked to communicate with an actor in this station. You have 7 minutes to complete the station.**

This station tests your ability to think logically and come up with a conclusion in the face of a new concept. Take your time to form your arguments for, and against the deterrent fees before speaking, so you avoid the common pitfall of stopping and starting your answer repeatedly.

As with any question where you have to form an opinion, a common format is to argue both sides of the argument, then present your personal opinion at the end.

- **Introduce yourself:** *"Hello, my name is Rahul, and I am a first-year medical student."*
- **Introduce the topic:** *"The NHS is under enormous financial pressure, and a deterrent fee is a mechanism to help reduce that burden."*
- **Present two to three points for the implementation of the fees.**
- **For example:** *"On one hand, implementing a deterrent fee could reduce the amount of self-limiting illnesses seen by the GPs, as patients are less likely to consult the GP for something small".*
- **Once you have presented your arguments, present your counterarguments:** *"However, implementing the fees could cause people to ignore potentially dangerous symptoms to save money."*
- **Another counterargument might be:** *"The fees may encourage more people to go to A&E rather than their GP, which would increase the already heavy burden on A&Es."*
- **To increase the validity of your points, supplement your argument by something highlighted by recent news:** *"Last winter, the majority of A&E trusts in the country did not reach their 4–hour targets regularly, and there were even reports of patients waiting inside ambulances for over an hour."*
- **Do not forget to come to a conclusion – this is your opinion, so there is no right or wrong answer:** *"Although I can appreciate why the deterrent fees may be a measure that would help save on costs, people already pay taxes to cover their health care. Incurring an additional cost seems excessive."*

14.16 (MMI) Describe the differences between the structure of the US and UK healthcare systems. In your answer, please refer to 'Obamacare' and how it will affect the US healthcare system. You have 2 minutes to prepare and 8 minutes to present your thoughts to the interviewer.

Private vs. public healthcare system

The key difference between both systems is the mix of private and public healthcare provision. According to the Commonwealth Fund in 2010, 56% of US citizens were covered by private health insurance, 27% were covered by public health programmes and the remaining 16% lacked health cover. In contrast, only approximately 11% of the UK population had private health insurance.

Structure of each healthcare system

The US healthcare system is made up of:

- *Payers* – includes individuals, insurance companies and public programmes. The public programmes are Medicare (distributed by federal government to those over 65 and disabled patients) and Medicaid (means-tested insurance distributed by states)
- *Providers* – all individuals and organisations that provide health care
- *Suppliers* – pharmaceutical and medical equipment companies
- *Consumers* – any person who seeks a healthcare service.

In the UK, the NHS comprises:

- *The Department of Health* – provides strategic leadership for public health, the NHS and social care in England. Aligns with government strategies via the Secretary of State for Health
- *Commissioners* – The Health and Social Care Act (2012) replaced Primary Care Trusts with Clinical Commissioning Groups (CCGs). CCGs are clinically led and responsive to local needs. They are charged with distributing a majority of the budget (£64 billion) to pay for healthcare services
- *Providers* – these are any willing supplier of NHS services, predominantly 'trusts'.

Healthcare spending

The USA spends 17% (£5950 per capita) of its GDP on healthcare, compared to the UK, which spends 9.1% (£2340 per capita) on its publicly funded system.

The Patient Protection and Affordable Care Act (2010), also known as *Obamacare*, aims to lower the price that the USA pays on healthcare. It requires all Americans to have health insurance, bans insurance companies from denying coverage to people with pre-existing health conditions and creates a fairer market place for insurance packages. In addition, the law allows young people to remain on their parents' plans until age 26, and expands eligibility for the government-run Medicaid health programme.

14.17 (T) There has been much recent press surrounding the change to the junior doctor contract. From your understanding, describe the main issues being disputed.

Over the last few years, the government has sought to instate a '7-day NHS' and reform the current contract for junior doctors. Despite two years of discussions, the BMA and government were unable to reach an agreement on the contract. In 2014 the government approached the Doctors' and Dentists' Review Body (DDRB) to lead on contract recommendations. Highlighted below are some of their recommendations under dispute:

- **Contractual safeguards:** the previous contract imposes a financial penalty on employers that regularly subject doctors to exhausting work patterns. The new contract recommends the maximum weekly hours be reduced to 72 from 91, and that doctors work no more than four days in a row. However, doctors suggest the new contract does not penalise employers adequately for non-compliant rotas. The BMA argues that this may result in overworked doctors, which is unsafe for patients.

- **Social hours definition and basic pay changes:** the DDRB recommendations will give doctors an increase of 11% in basic salary. However, there is a change in unsocial hours pay. The new contract seeks to extend standard working hours from 60 to 90 hours overall. Standard time, currently 7 am to 7 pm Monday to Friday, would be changed to 7 am to 10 pm Monday to Saturday. The BMA argues that this means some doctors will face a pay cut of up to 30% based on the hours worked, is detrimental to sleep patterns and will result in a dysfunctional work/life balance.

- **Pay progression:** the new contract will aim to tie pay progression with experience and training grade, rather than years worked in post. This is potentially a huge hit for those who take time out of training to have children, or pursue academic research.

These are just some of the key proposed changes in the new contract; make sure you familiarise yourself with other points by looking at the BMA, and NHS Employers websites. For each of these issues, as discussed above, think about their implications for doctors, patients and the NHS. This is meant to provide a background to the dispute, but it is important to familiarise yourself with plans for a 7-day NHS and the other current issues facing the NHS.

Chapter 15 | Technical skills questions

15.1 *(MMI) You are a medical student on placement in a GP practice, where you see Mr Evans who tripped and fell on his walk to the local shop this morning. His right wrist is very painful and he is worried that it might be broken. The GP suggests that he attends A&E for X-rays but asks you to put Mr Evans' arm in a sling to make him more comfortable in the meantime. Please put Mr Evans' arm in a triangular bandage sling. A student will demonstrate how to do this before you meet Mr Evans for 3 minutes and you will then have 5 minutes to put the arm in the sling.*

The interviewer will be assessing how well you communicate with Mr Evans whilst demonstrating the skill.

Introduction
- Introduce yourself: *"Hello Mr Evans. My name is Noushin Askari, I am one of the medical students working at the practice".*
- Explain what you are going to do: *"The doctor has asked me to put your arm in a sling. This will help support your wrist and make you more comfortable until you can be seen in A&E."*
- Gain consent: *"Is this OK with you?"*
- Build rapport: *"Please let me know if you are uncomfortable at any point and I will stop."*

Skill
- Ensure that you have the correct wrist.
- Place Mr Evans' arm in the triangular bandage as demonstrated to you previously. (You can find videos of how to do this easily online, should you wish to practise this station 'for real'.)
- Be careful when moving the arm, since the wrist may be broken and you may hurt Mr Evans.
- If you sense that Mr Evans is in pain, stop what you are doing and check that he is OK!

Conclusion
- Thank Mr Evans: *"Thank you for letting me put on the sling. I hope it helps your wrist feel more comfortable".*
- Make sure Mr Evans knows what to do next and direct him to A&E if necessary.

15.2 (MMI) Describe what you see in this photograph. (A photograph of a 'lesion' [e.g. an ulcer] will be displayed). You have 3 minutes to review the photograph and then 4 minutes to describe it to the interviewer.

This interview station is a test of communication skills and being able to think on your feet. You may be required to present your answer to the interviewer (or to write your answer on a piece of paper, in which case make sure your handwriting is legible!) The interviewers will not expect you to be able to make a diagnosis or use the technical terms used by doctors, but a lot of information can be conveyed using simple descriptions. The key is to try to imagine you are giving the description over the phone and try to give a description detailed enough for the person at the other end of the phone to be able to draw it. Below are some of the main points to consider:

Patient: the age and/or sex of the patient are worth mentioning although this may only be possible if the photo shows a facial lesion or a genital/ breast lesion. Try to mention the race of the patient or their skin tone: these can be important since some conditions are more common in some ethnicities than others.

Skin condition: remember the abbreviation SSSECC, as this can help you to cover all the elements:

- *Site* (e.g. right hand, left side of nose) – saying where the 'lesion' is sounds obvious but can be difficult if the image is very zoomed in. Think about whether it might be in a sun-exposed area or on the inside/outside of a joint.
- *Size* – there may be a ruler in the image to help you, otherwise you may have to try to estimate from other features in the photograph.
- *Shape and symmetry* – time to use some descriptive language. It may be a simple shape such as circular or ovoid but may be very irregular and asymmetrical.
- *Edge* – is the edge of the lesion well demarcated or is it blurry?
- *Colour* – there are technical terms for certain colours such as erythematous (red) but don't be afraid to use the simple terms such as red, purple, black, green, yellow, etc. Be sure to mention if there are multiple colours. If a lesion is more 'tanned' like a freckle this is described as 'pigmented', and if the skin is lighter than normal it is said to be 'de-pigmented'.
- *Contour* – this may be difficult to gauge from a photo but think about whether the lesion looks flat, raised or sunken.

15.3 **(MMI) Memorise this picture. You will then be asked to describe it to the interviewer in as much detail as possible. [A photograph e.g. of a city skyline will be shown]. You have 3 minutes to review the picture and 4 minutes to describe it to the interviewer.**

This task is both a test of memory and a test of accurate communication. It may seem abstract but is a very good way to test how well you will be able to communicate information on a telephone, e.g. describing a fracture you see on an X-ray to your consultant who is answering the telephone from home and can't see the X-ray for him- or herself.

The process of memorisation is very personal and can easily be practised by describing random photos to a friend who has to draw the image you describe.

You may find it helpful to divide the picture into more bite-size chunks (e.g. divide the picture into four). Alternatively you may find it easier to focus on the most striking feature and then remember everything relative to that. Whichever technique you use, experiment and practise until you are happy.

When looking at the picture and then describing it, begin with the most basic features (e.g. the picture is a landscape photo of a city skyline, with the tallest buildings roughly in the middle). Then systematically work through the finer details of the image.

Keep an eye on the time to make sure you don't neglect certain areas of the picture.

15.4 *(MMI) The person in the station you are about to enter is totally deaf. They have not used lace-up shoes before. Your instructions are to demonstrate to them how to tie their shoelaces using whatever method you deem appropriate. You have 7 minutes to complete this station.*

This station is an extremely challenging one, and is typical of some of the newer MMI stations that are entering widespread use within some universities. Challenging communication scenarios such as these are encountered daily by staff in the health service, and excellent communication skills are a must for all doctors. This station will assess your ability to remain patient in a potentially frustrating scenario, and to remain empathetic with the actor. It is important not to appear rushed or frustrated at any stage. In everyday clinical practice, an interpreter would be provided in cases such as this, but this has been made deliberately more challenging to push your communication skills to the limit!

An effective way to approach this scenario would be as follows:
- Enter the room and greet the actor with a warm smile and offer a handshake. Given the existing barrier to communication, the maintenance of eye contact assumes even greater importance than normal here.
- In order to demonstrate this skill, it is important to work through it very slowly and methodically, ensuring the actor has a good view of your hands throughout. It would be a good idea to take your own shoe off, or use one provided (it is more likely that one will be provided) and place it on your knee, so the actor can have a clearer view of it.
- Break the tying of the shoelaces down into small stages, with deliberate, clear hand movements. After each stage, check that the actor has understood the stage involved by making eye contact with them.
- After you have demonstrated the entire skill, gesture with an open hand towards the shoe, or hand the shoe to the actor, in order to indicate that they should attempt it.
- The actor will doubtless be briefed to deliberately make mistakes when attempting to tie the laces – the interviewers will be carefully viewing your response to this! At no stage appear frustrated, and simply return to the previous stage performed correctly, and demonstrate the skill from there, until the actor manages it.
- Check understanding using clear gestures and eye contact throughout and remain positive and encouraging throughout the station.

15.5 **(MMI) You have come across a person collapsed on the street. They appear to have a leg injury and are confused. Demonstrate what you will do. You will be asked to communicate with an actor in this station. You have 7 minutes to complete the station.**

- **Introduce yourself to the patient.** Speak loudly to ensure the patient hears. *"Hello, my name is Kate. Are you all right?"*
- **The patient responds** by mumbling that they have fallen over.
- There is a phone nearby. Explain to the patient that you are going to **call an ambulance**.
- Mimic dialling an emergency number, and **asking for help**: *"Hello, I would like an ambulance please. A female, age 20–30, has collapsed on Marylebone Road."*
- **Return to the patient.**
- **Reassure** them that help is on its way.
- If there is some sort of gauze or clean cloth nearby, you may attempt to **stem blood flow from their leg**. Explain clearly to the patient what you are doing and be sure to receive consent before you touch them.
- **Comfort the patient**, who is understandably distressed: *"The ambulance will be here soon. I am here to help."*
- Try to gain as much information as possible about their injuries, so that you can explain it to the paramedics when they arrive: *"Has this happened before?"* or *"Do you know why you collapsed?"*

At your level, this station is testing how you communicate with a distressed individual, while remaining calm and in control of the situation. It is also testing basic technical skills, like using the apparatus available for calling the ambulance and stopping blood loss.

15.6 (MMI) This is a skills station. Please read the instructions below carefully. Follow the instructions and complete the tasks within 5 minutes. The interviewer will observe your actions only and will not be able to provide any extra information.

Instructions:

1. Wash your hands and put a pair of size-appropriate gloves on.

2. Identify the toothed forceps (see photo) among these surgical instruments.

3. Using the toothed forceps, pick up the suture as demonstrated in the photo.

4. Dispose of suture in the yellow sharps bin.

5. Remove gloves and dispose of them appropriately in the bin provided.

This is a very simple station, but one in which students find themselves making silly mistakes by not reading the instructions carefully. There can be a great many variations on the content of the station but your ability to follow instructions clearly will be the common theme.

TOP TIP Candidates often rush into this station because they feel like they are short on time. The reality is that candidates have more than enough time and should finish with minutes to spare. Do not start this station before you have read the instructions at least twice.

The following errors are very common in stations like the one described above and will lead to failure of the station:

- The candidate fails to wash their hands. Even if there is no soap, water or hand sanitiser available, stating that you would wash your hands will still impress.
- The candidate fails to put gloves on.
- The candidate does not identify the correct type of forceps.
- The candidate does not dispose of the suture in the correct bin. There may be a blue, yellow and red bin in front of you, and choosing the correct one will be vital when you are a doctor.

TOP TIP If you make a mistake during the station, you should revert to the instructions to amend your mistake and avoid panicking. If the mistake cannot be amended, complete the station as best you can and wait for the next station. If your mistake cannot be undone then acknowledging that you have made a mistake and explaining to the examiner what you should have done, may be a good plan.

15.7 **(MMI) You are provided with a child's playmat. On the playmat are aerial pictures of shops and a network of roads. You are also provided with a small toy car. Your interviewer will be blindfolded and you will be asked to guide him around the road from the train station to the post office using only words. You will not be allowed to touch the map, the car or the interviewer's hand during the interview. You have 5 minutes.**

This scenario is analogous to a doctor (you) communicating with a patient (the interviewer) whilst the patient is suffering some level of stress (blindfolded). This is a test of pure communication. Use the following steps to help you:

Introduction

Introduce yourself and explain your role. Ask the interviewer their name. Gain permission to use their name: *"Hello, my name is Mitchell Turnock. I am here to guide you around the map, from the train station to the post office. Can I ask for your name please? May I call you _____?"*

Perception

This is where you build rapport with the interviewer to gain trust. Building trust is very important here. With trust and clear instruction, this task will run smoothly. This is also an opportunity to show empathy. Use it well:

> *"I see you are wearing a blindfold. How does that feel?"*
> *"How much do you know about the task at hand?"*

Gauging how much the interviewer knows and how confident they are about the task is crucial. It will guide your instructions.

Explanation

Explain the task and the rules to the interviewer. Ask if they understand. Ask if they have any questions.

Instruct

Give very clear, unambiguous instructions:

> *"Move the car forward until I say stop. When I say stop, please stop immediately."*
> *"Turn left."*
> *"Move slowly backwards slightly further until I say stop."*

If the interviewer makes a mistake, and they invariably will to test you, say, *"stop"* and stay very calm and empathetic, e.g. *"It must be very difficult using just me to guide you."*

Close

"You have arrived at the post office. Thank you. How clear did you find my instructions?"

Chapter 16 | Thinking on your feet

16.1 *(T) Give an example of a situation when you have supported a friend in a difficult social circumstance. What issues did you face and how did you help them?*

This question is looking for a specific situation. Prior to the interview it is a good idea to think of a few scenarios that you could use for different questions. Try to use your feelings to make the answer sound individual and genuine. You can answer using the 'BARL' technique that you learnt about in *Question 3.3*: **B**ackground, **A**ction, **R**esult and **L**ink to medicine:

Background
"The mother of one of my friends was diagnosed with ovarian cancer last year. It was a shock to everyone as she was always so fit and healthy. It was a very difficult time for my friend and her family and it put a lot of strain on them. Fortunately, I have never had something like this happen to me so at first I found it hard to relate to the situation. I knew my friend was finding it very difficult so I did my best to comfort and support her. I spent a lot of time with her and tried to take her mind off it by taking her out and talking about positive things."

Action
"I offered her support when she went to visit her mother in hospital and sat and chatted with her family and mother for hours. I could tell her mother was scared but we all reassured her that the doctors were doing everything they could. By visiting her we offered her some happiness and my friend said that she couldn't have done it without me."

Result
"I knew she really appreciated me being there and felt that I had helped her through a difficult time and that my support had made a real difference. Others tell me I am a caring and compassionate person and I think this truly facilitated the situation."

This question offers you a chance to show off your personal attributes. Saying *"Others tell me I am a caring and compassionate person..."* is a good way of objectively publicising your strengths, without sounding boastful. You have then backed these strengths up by showing how you used them in a situation to overcome problems.

Link to medicine
This situation demonstrates my ability to empathise with others and to communicate in a sensitive manner. These are key skills required by doctors.

> **TOP TIP** Don't worry if the scenario is mundane; it is how you dealt with it that is important. You want to show the interviewer that you are supportive and empathetic and can deal with difficult situations with a sensible approach.

16.2 (T) Give an example of a time when you have had to show empathy.

Empathy is the ability to put yourself in someone else's shoes and to share their experiences and feelings so that you can understand how it would feel to be in their position. Empathy is a vital skill for all doctors and is a major focus during medical school.

For this answer you want to choose a specific example rather than vaguely talking about how you always show empathy to your friends and family. Try not to make things up, as it is easy to trip up when you are nervous and the interviewer will see straight through it. Also it is harder to talk passionately about something that isn't real.

Make the answer personal by talking about what you did, how it made you feel and what the final outcome was for you. It would be helpful to think of some examples to questions like this before you go into the interview so that you have a few scenarios that can be adapted to address a variety of questions. It is useful to also answer these questions with a structure, e.g. '**BARL**': **B**ackground, **A**ction, **R**esult and **L**ink to medicine (see *Question 3.3* for more details):

Background: Frame the situation you were in.
"Recently, I have been volunteering with disabled children. I have been caring for one child in particular for a few weeks and have developed a strong bond with her. She is wheelchair-bound and needs help with feeding. We were on a day trip to the zoo and some children sitting on the opposite table to us were staring at her and laughing while I was trying to feed her."

Action: What did you do?
"This was a difficult situation as it was obviously very upsetting for the young girl and it was also an eye-opener for me to see the harsh reality of it. I sensed through her body language that she was about to cry so I decided we should leave the table and eat somewhere else. I tried to imagine how she must feel having to deal with being in a wheelchair and also having people judging her all the time."

Result: What happened because of your actions?
"Afterwards we spoke about what had happened and she opened up to me. I comforted her and explained that I was always there if she ever wanted to talk. By putting myself in her shoes, it helped me to understand how difficult it must be and I was able to support her better. She seemed much happier and I felt I had really made a difference by just taking the time to speak to her about how she felt."

Link: Relate the example you have given back to medicine.
"Empathy is a great quality to possess and is essential for all doctors. It is a personal attribute that I believe I possess and I am continually developing."

16.3 (T) Give an example of a time when you have played an effective role in a team.

It is essential to be able to work successfully both within a team and as a team leader. Choose an example that shows that you are versatile and have all aspects of a good team player. It may be a good idea to identify some points that make you a good team player and remember to incorporate them into your answer. Don't forget that using a structure can help in your answer, e.g. '**BARL**': **B**ackground, **A**ction, **R**esult and **L**ink to medicine:

Positive team–playing skills:
- Treat other team members with respect and encourage them to participate
- Take into consideration the opinions of others
- Recognise your role (strengths and weaknesses) and others' roles within a team
- Versatile and open-minded
- Willing to consider others' opinions
- Willing to help and pull your weight, especially if someone is struggling
- Communication and listening skills
- Reliable and motivated.

Background
"I was a team member in a hiking expedition with my school through the mountains. We had a team member who seemed very weary and was slowing down dramatically in their walking speed."

Action
"I perceived that they were really struggling with exhaustion and asked if they were OK. When they told me they weren't I raised this point with the rest of the team on their behalf, showing that I was willing to take into consideration their feelings. I asked if the others might be happy to help out and asked if my friend Tom, who was an excellent map-reader, could suggest a more direct route. This demonstrates that I am versatile. I also offered to carry some of the heavier items in their rucksack for a while to give them some rest, demonstrating that I pull my weight on behalf of the team."

Result
"We reached our campsite slightly earlier due to a more direct route, and my friend was able to get some good rest that evening before completing the full hike the following day. They remained passionate about hiking and went on to become leader of the hiking club at school."

Link to medicine
"My communication skills, versatility, empathy and motivation skills will be very useful should I be fortunate enough to work in a medical team."

16.4 (MMI) You are called to see a patient who is bleeding profusely from a large wound. They are becoming critically ill because of the bleeding. You know they have HIV. There are no gloves available. What do you do? What are the issues here?

This question is testing your ability to think on your feet when faced with a challenge in the hospital environment.

You could begin with your course of action but show that you are being thoughtful. You should demonstrate:

- **That your safety and the safety of the patient are of utmost priority**

"Though the risk of infection may be relatively low, I am aware that my own safety is very important and this may impact on the safety of other patients if I become infected. I am also aware that the patient is in a critically ill situation and needs urgent help – this is of extreme importance. Throughout this scenario I would communicate clearly with the patient."

- **That you have problem-solving skills**

"I would ask for urgent help from colleagues. I would ask the nursing staff if they had a spare supply of gloves in a cupboard/on the emergency trolley or whether they had any alternative types of gloves (e.g. the sterile ones they use for procedures)."

Note the interviewer may say, "None of these are available" at this stage – this is common. They are simply pushing you to see what else you would do and to assess your problem-solving skills further.

"I could ask if someone had suitable protection to assist with the patient (maybe already wearing gloves but they were unused?) or I could call a colleague to assist while I get a pair of gloves from a nearby ward. If none of these were an option I might be able to use something else to put pressure on the wound, such as asking the patient, instead of me, to press very hard on it with the dressing. I would also like to get some urgent senior help."

- **That you have a desire to improve things for the future**

"This scenario raises some questions, such as why there were no gloves on the ward. I would work with senior colleagues to ensure this didn't happen again, perhaps by offering to work with the senior doctors and nurses on the equipment ordering procedures at the hospital."

16.5 (T) Tell me about a challenge you have faced and how you overcame it.

This is a broad and quite common question. The interviewers want to see how well you can apply your problem-solving skills as well as testing important qualities they are looking for in a medical student, such as ability to cope with pressure and stress and be resilient. You may want to use the 'BARL' approach: **B**ackground, **A**ction, **R**esult and **L**ink to medicine.

The example doesn't have to be work- or study-related but can also be drawn from extra-curricular activities. Examples could include a fundraising task, a project that did not go to plan, unexpected extra responsibility or a family problem, or something more general such as balancing a substantial commitment alongside your studies (such as a job or a sport). Once you have chosen your example, break it down. You may want to follow the steps below when formatting your answer:

Background: Why was it difficult?
e.g. *"During my final year of A levels, a significant challenge for me was my mother experiencing an illness during my exams. I initially found it quite difficult to juggle schoolwork along with other new responsibilities such as taking care of my brother during her recovery, but I persevered."*

Action: What **practical** steps did you take to overcome it?
e.g. *"I aimed to deal with this through effective time management and asking for support when required. I motivated myself to keep going by remaining positive throughout, creating a revision plan with timed deadlines and when I did become overwhelmed, I took a step back and kept the situation in perspective."*

Result: What was the result?
e.g. *"I was able to succeed in my forthcoming exams and gained A, A, B grades. As a result, I learnt a great deal about perseverance and discipline. I also learnt more about myself in the process, such as my ability to adapt to new and unexpected situations whilst remaining determined."*

Link to medicine: How might this help you as a doctor?
You might want to add in the keywords of key personality traits that are important as a doctor such as: *resilience, discipline, challenge* and *perseverance*.

16.6 **(MMI) You are asked to discuss with a patient who tells you that he is not going to tell his girlfriend that he is HIV positive. Please discuss with the patient (actor) and explain what your course of action will be. You have 10 minutes.**

This is a difficult situation. The patient is understandably worried that his girlfriend may reject him, but by not telling her he puts her at risk of HIV. It is important to speak to the patient calmly and without judgment to encourage him to protect his girlfriend from harm. Berating and scolding the patient is unlikely to work. However, the patient needs to understand the seriousness of the situation. The patient may have only recently found out that he is HIV positive and may still be coming to terms with the implications of the diagnosis for himself, let alone another person.

An appropriate approach to the situation would be:

- **Start by introducing yourself:** *"Hello, my name is Wang Xiu Lan, I am one of the doctors working at the clinic. I have been asked to talk to you about your recent diagnosis."*
- **Ask how he is and how he is coping with his diagnosis:** *"How are you feeling? It must be difficult coming to terms with the diagnosis."*
- **Let them know that as part of the counselling process you need to discuss minimising the risk of transmission to others:** *"As part of the HIV counselling service we need to talk about minimising the risk of transmitting the disease to others."*
- **Ask if he currently has a sexual partner:** *"I understand that you have a girlfriend?"*
- **Has he thought about how the diagnosis might affect the relationship:** *"Have you considered how the diagnosis might affect your relationship?"*
- **Let him know he must use condoms to prevent transmission.**
- Inform him that he will need to notify past and present partners so that they can be tested themselves.
- If he is unhappy to do this himself, the clinic can notify his girlfriend that she may be at risk of HIV and invite her in for testing.
- **Let the patient know that letting his girlfriend know is the right thing to do.**

If all attempts to encourage the patient to tell his girlfriend fail then you would be justified to share information without his consent, as this would be considered to be in the public interest. You must inform the patient if you are going to break confidentiality for this purpose. You would notify his girlfriend that she may have been exposed to HIV and invite her to attend for a test.

16.7 (T) The government wants to implement compulsory school dinners for all primary school children. Weigh up the pros and cons, and give your opinion on this.

The interviewers are looking at your ability to take unfamiliar scenarios and talk about them in a balanced way.

Start off with the benefits of compulsory school meals:
- Providing well-balanced, nutritious meals to all children can help tackle childhood obesity
- Equality in dining experience for all students irrespective of socioeconomic background
- Cheaper for parents who may have struggled to pay for packed lunches.

Now talk about the disadvantages, offering solutions if possible:
- Children have different dietary requirements, and this will need to be taken into consideration, e.g. halal/kosher meat, vegetarian/vegan options, food allergies, medical conditions such as coeliac disease, patients with cystic fibrosis may require a greater calorific intake, etc.
- May put a financial burden on schools, and they may need to hire more staff for the kitchen. Indeed the dining room may not be large enough to cater for all students.
- May not be a wise use of money – would it be better spent on means-tested school lunches, whereby those who need them most receive them, whilst those who can afford to purchase lunch are asked to provide their own?

End with your opinion
Now that you have gone into detail about the pros and cons of implementing such a scheme you can give your opinion on the matter, e.g.:
"Although there might be some difficulties in implementing compulsory school dinners to all children, I believe that such a scheme is a big step forward in tackling some key issues affecting children, such as childhood obesity which could lead to a lifetime of problems."

16.8 (T) A patient has come to you for an abortion but this goes against your strong religious beliefs. What do you do?

Even if you have not read the GMC guidelines on this scenario, you should be able to use your common sense to find a suitable solution to your problem.

While this question may be handled in a couple of different ways what you must not say is that you would deny the patient treatment.

You would first need to talk to the patient and elicit a few important details before you continue.
You need to know how old the patient is. If the patient is a minor, the scenario will completely change, as there are many other aspects to consider. Therefore, mention to the panel that you would like to rule this out.

Another thing you would need to find out from the patient is how many weeks pregnant they are. Under the current UK law, an abortion can only be performed during the first 24 weeks of pregnancy. It is only permissible after this cut-off if there is a substantial risk to the baby or mother's life.

You need to assess the mental capacity of the patient to ensure the patient is fully aware of the risks of the procedure.

Current legislation requires two doctors to agree to the abortion in a non-emergency setting.

What can you do next?
It is within your rights as a doctor to not perform (or even make a decision on) an abortion if you are not comfortable with it, but you cannot prevent the patient from having an abortion. Therefore once you have established that the patient fits the criteria, you must refer the patient on to a colleague who will be able to make a decision upon whether the abortion is appropriate or not.

The law in Northern Ireland
The 1967 Abortion Act does not extend to Northern Ireland, where the law remains as it was in the rest of the UK prior to the 1967 Act. In Northern Ireland an abortion can only be performed if a doctor is acting to save the life of the mother or if continuing the pregnancy would result in the mother becoming a "mental or physical wreck". There is ongoing debate about the law in Northern Ireland and it is worth checking the current status of the debate before your interview.

16.9 (T) Give me an example of a time when you appropriately stood up to someone in a position of authority. Is it right that the medical profession is arranged in a hierarchical fashion?

This question is included to ascertain if you are a person who speaks up for what is right, and would be willing to speak up if they believed that patient safety was being compromised. The author of the Francis report published another report in February 2015, entitled *Freedom to Speak Up*, in which one of his recommendations was the fostering of a culture where all members of staff can speak up about concerns that they have.

Speaking up can be a difficult thing to do. An appropriate example answer is provided below:

"During a training session for the school soccer team, I noticed that the team captain was being unfairly and publicly critical of one of the other players on the team, and that he had been behaving like this for a few weeks. After the training session had ended, I asked to speak with the captain, and asked him why he was treating the other player in this way. I sensitively told him that I thought his behaviour was unacceptable, and that if it continued I would have to broach the topic with the coach."

This example demonstrates a proportional approach, with a plan if your actions do not resolve the problem.

With regard to the follow-on question about the hierarchical arrangement of medicine, it is important to provide the pros and cons of this arrangement, and that you have come to a considered conclusion:

Pros of hierarchical arrangement:

- More senior doctors have more extensive training and experience than their more junior colleagues, and it is right that they ultimately make decisions regarding patient care.
- Junior doctors should always know who to go to for guidance when they are uncertain.
- The training of junior doctors by consultants allows them to benefit from the experience of their senior colleagues.

Cons of hierarchical arrangement:

- Junior members of staff may feel it is not their place to speak up when they have identified a problem with patient care.
- It may contribute to making senior doctors less approachable for patients, and they may keep some of their concerns to themselves as a result.
- There are interdisciplinary hierarchies that can lead to some members of the healthcare team feeling less valued. Moreover, there is a risk that essential aspects of patient care that these healthcare professionals represent can receive less attention as a result.

16.10   (T) Is medicine an art or a science?

The phrase 'evidence-based medicine' is a guiding principle of modern Western medicine, dictating that all care must have a scientific basis. Despite this guiding principle, anyone who has ever required medical assistance, or witnessed good medical practice up close, will acknowledge that it is the 'human' side that makes a real difference to patients and their families. The art of medicine is in the application of sound scientific theory, using it to heal patients' bodies, minds and souls.

This blend of art and science is what sets medicine apart from pure scientific disciplines and the arts, requiring applicants to medical school to demonstrate ability in both fields. With this in mind, prior to your interview you should ensure that your achievements, experience and interests cover the spectrum between arts and sciences, rather than clustering towards just one extreme.

Should one feel like demonstrating a passion for debating controversial topics, or indeed simply want to broaden the conversation, it is possible to argue that medicine is becoming more scientific. Background reading of the mainstream press should keep you abreast of the biggest medical breakthroughs as you prepare for your interview – there can be no doubt that scientific advances are very rapidly followed by medical leaps forward. At the same time some feel that healthcare is becoming too scientific and driven by numbers – perhaps what is required is a re-calibration towards more humanity in medicine.

16.11 *(MMI) There's a runaway train about to hit five people. You can switch the signals at a junction and it will take a different path, killing one person. What do you do? Would you change your mind if you found out all five people were murderers? You have 10 minutes to discuss your thoughts with an interviewer.*

With any ethical question you face at a medical school interview, you should focus on showing your ability to reason. Whilst it is not necessary to firmly adopt a side during a question such as this, you should be able to defend any position you take with sound reason and be able to partially consider both sides of the argument.

Perhaps equally importantly, be structured in your answer. Do not just churn out lots of various points without expanding on them, but give perhaps one or two answers for both sides and be able to enter into a discussion with the interviewer as necessary.

There are many stances you could take when answering this question. One issue that could be discussed is whether as a human, with inbuilt morals, there is a difference between being active in the event (i.e. switching the signals) and being involved in saving five people but killing one, or being passive in the event (i.e. not switching the signals) and not playing a part in the deaths of five people. Many would argue that people have certain duties and that once it is accepted to make such a decision, as in this case, there is no case for inaction.

Another area you may wish to discuss is for those who chose to save five lives, do they do this as five lives lost is worse than one life lost if all lives are considered equal (termed consequentialist) or have they intended to save five lives and that is the only moral consideration (termed intentionalist)?

Certainly, when approaching the second part of this question, a consequentialist approach may be important: are the lives of murderers worth less than the lives of innocents? Does one even start to consider the potential further lives lost if the murderers are saved and they then go on to commit further murders, equating to more lives lost?

A favourable answer here would be to say all lives are equal and then enter into a healthy discussion with the interviewer on this point.

Do not be fazed by any ethical question such as this. Even if you do not understand some of the more complex ethical arguments (the thoughts described above are to pose possible discussion points you may wish to raise), be structured in your answer and be prepared to discuss any points you make further with the interviewer.

16.12   *(T) You come across a house on fire as you walk down a rural road. There are people trapped in the house and the fire service has been called, yet will not arrive for another hour and you are the only one around who can help those inside. Who would you save in the fire: someone with the cure to cancer or your own father?*

As with any ethical question such as this, it is important to give a considered and honest answer. Whilst this may seem like quite a far-fetched scenario, it can be translated to many common parts of modern medicine, including ethical issues involving medically treating your own relatives or the allocation of resources within healthcare.

Providing a good answer to this will show the interviewer you can be thoughtful and critical towards an important topic that many clinicians face every day. With these types of questions, be structured with your answer and be able to expand on any points the interviewer challenges you with. Remember, there is not necessarily a right or wrong answer to this, but you should show a good understanding of both sides of the argument and form a balanced and considered opinion.

There are a few topics you could discuss with such a question:
Firstly, take the impact that each man has. A man who has the cure to cancer has the potential to save thousands of lives, an obvious answer. However, he is likely to work in a team on this cure, with the work backed up and saved elsewhere, not being the sole individual working on that project. One could argue that this man has no more individual potential to save lives than your otherwise 'unskilled' father. Therefore, does the personal impact your father has actually mean that you should save your father?

Another angle that could be discussed is to consider what your father tells you to do. Assuming in this scenario you have the time to discuss such a decision with both men, being able to discuss the situation with your father may relieve some of the emotional pressure on the scenario, if your father does decide to heroically sacrifice himself.

Perhaps you take a passive role in proceedings and don't save either man, as you do not want to be actively involved in the other man's death. Many may disagree with such a viewpoint but it is certainly an area for fruitful discussion.

A final discussion point may be how to value one individual's life over another. Your father may have his own set of skills that can benefit individuals in other ways, not just scientific skills. Are there other areas you must look at when valuing a life and an individual's skill set is not solely important? The quantification of the value of human life is certainly an interesting area that you may wish to discuss.

As alluded to, for this interview station, there may not necessarily be a right or wrong answer. Instead, you should form logical arguments for both sides of the discussion and be prepared to defend any statements you do make.

16.13 **(MMI) You are a newly qualified doctor and a couple you have known for a number of years recently had their first child. This baby was born with significant health problems, for which a kidney transplant is required. No matches have been found for the transplant so they are planning on having another child so that they can use an organ to save their newborn's life. What do you think about children being born for their organs to match another child who needs them? You have 7 minutes to discuss with the interviewer.**

As with any interview question that has an ethical component to it, you should be forming arguments for both sides of the discussion and be able to expand any points further with the examiner. You may decide to come down on one side or the other in your answer, but be prepared to defend your answer from questioning; do not be put off if you are asked difficult questions as it is likely that the interviewer is trying to push you further in the debate.

There are several ways in which you could approach this question and it is not possible to cover all of them. However, aspects you may want to consider include:

Pros:

- One life saved outweighs all other outcomes. An individual can survive with only one kidney, so whilst the firstborn survives, the second child will also lead an unaffected life, with the added bonus that the firstborn's life has been saved.
- People have the right to (and do) bring babies into the world for no pre-determined reason at all. If parents love and raise a child well, then the reasoning of conception almost becomes irrelevant: existing is better than not existing.

Cons:

- How will the child react if they find out they were brought into the world to serve such a purpose? Regardless of the amount of love they received from the parents, knowing that they were brought into the world not due to a parental want, but to save their elder sibling, could be argued to cause significant psychological effects on the younger sibling.
- Can the parents say it is really in the best interest of a child who will likely not be able to understand the risks of the procedure? The child will not have the capacity to make such a decision for itself and it is down to the parents to make that decision for them. However, it may turn out that as the second child grows up they do not agree with the fact they lost a kidney to their elder sibling.

These are just a few areas you may wish to explore in your discussion. Be structured in both sides of your response and be able to discuss and defend any points you make.

16.14   *(MMI) You are a first-year medical student living in university accommodation. You notice cuts on the wrists of your friend, who lives with you. Discuss this situation with the friend, who will be played by an actor, in a manner you deem appropriate. You have 7 minutes to complete this station.*

Doctors often have to intervene to help colleagues they feel may be struggling, and it is important to do so in a sensitive, compassionate manner. This situation is analogous to being asked to provide support for a struggling colleague, and represents an opportunity to demonstrate empathy and altruism. An appropriate way to approach it would be as follows:

- Ask to speak with your friend in private, in a place where they will feel comfortable.
- Give your friend an opportunity to speak, and to discuss anything they want to by asking a very open question to begin with *"How have you been getting on recently?"*
- Your friend may reveal that they have been in difficulty recently, and if they do, remain empathetic and use phrases such as *"I understand that must be very difficult for you"*. It would be a bad idea to say "I know how you feel", as in all likelihood you don't, and your friend may respond badly to this phrase.
- If they are not immediately forthcoming about what has been troubling them, it would be appropriate to gently enquire as to what is wrong, as you have noticed cuts on their wrist *"I was wondering if everything was all right with you? I noticed some cuts on your wrist"*.
- Listen actively to what your friend is telling you, maintaining eye contact and nodding appropriately. Let what they have to say come to a natural pause, without interrupting them.
- Try to explore potential reasons for why they might be feeling low: Are they struggling with their course? Have they had difficulties in their personal life? Do they have financial concerns?
- It would be a good idea to try to help them find a solution to their problems: helping them with a study plan if they are struggling with their workload, or offering to help them to budget if they have financial issues. However, avoid being caught in the middle of a personal dispute if there is one.
- It would be important here to demonstrate your knowledge of sources of help for people with issues such as this: the university counselling service, their own GP, the Samaritans. Offer to come with them to an appointment with the counsellor or GP if they feel they couldn't face this on their own.
- Thank your friend for speaking to you. Tell them they can come to you at any time with any problems they have.

16.15 **(MMI) You are a doctor working on the intensive care unit ward. A child has been declared brain-dead, but the parents refuse to allow you to remove the life support machine. Another child coming out of surgery has need for the ITU bed. Explain this issue to the bed manager, who will be played by an actor, and explain what your next action is and why. You have 7 minutes.**

This is an extremely challenging and complicated scenario. There are several aspects being tested:
- **Communication** – you must recall all the facts you have just learned and relay them accurately to the bed manager.
- **Empathy** – the parents of the brain-dead child are understandably distraught and require sympathy and consideration.
- **Ability to cope under pressure** – it is an emotional situation, one that requires clear and logical thinking to achieve the best possible outcome.

A model answer may be:
- **Introduce yourself**: *"Hello, my name is Paul, and I am one of the doctors working on ITU."*
- **Take your time to explain the situation clearly**: *"We need to find an ITU bed for a patient coming out of surgery. Currently, on one bed, there is a brain-dead patient, but his parents do not want him removed from the life support machine."*
- **Make an attempt to find a solution that would suit both parties**: *"I will ask the consultant if there is any other patient on ITU who is suitable to go to a lower dependency ward, to make space for our surgical patient."*
- **Address the distraught parents**: *"If we could help the parents come to terms with their son's condition, we could remove him from the life support machine with their consent."*
- **Demonstrate empathy**: *"They are understandably distressed and need kindness and understanding at this hard time. We may have to explain the implications of our surgical patient if he does not get care in the intensive care unit."*

This is an extremely distressing question to be asked, but it has been asked before. Try not to jump to the hasty conclusion of 'turning the switch off' for the brain-dead child. After all, you have five to seven minutes to answer this question. It is much more important that you discuss the situation, and emotions of the parties involved, then come to a conclusion.

16.16 (MMI) You see one of your medical student colleagues taking photographs of a patient using their smartphone as you walk on to the ward. You decide to intervene. The interviewer will play the medical student and you have to interact with them. You have 7 minutes to complete this station.

This is a challenging scenario. It requires you to use sensitivity.

An example way to tackle the situation might be:

- **Introduce yourself** to the medical student and to the patient, if they are still with the patient.
- Ask if it is OK to have a quiet word with the student away from the bedside. **Take the student away from the patient** to avoid making a scene.
- **Enquire** what they were doing when they were with the patient. Was it, in fact, a scenario where the student was looking up some facts on their phone or emailing their tutor? Or were they definitely taking photographs?
- **Explain that you believe you saw them** taking photographs of a patient.
- **Recommend they stop** what they are doing and **delete** immediately any pictures taken.
- **Recommend that they apologise to, and be honest with the patient** about what has happened.
- **Explain that they should agree to discuss this with their supervisor or mentor.** If they refuse then gently and tactfully explain that you would have to do so if they didn't, since it is a serious breach of patient confidentiality.